10-MINUTES SCIATICA EXERCISES FOR SENIORS

Simple and effective home treatment Exercises for Lasting Relief

Charles K Benavides

TABLE OF CONTENT

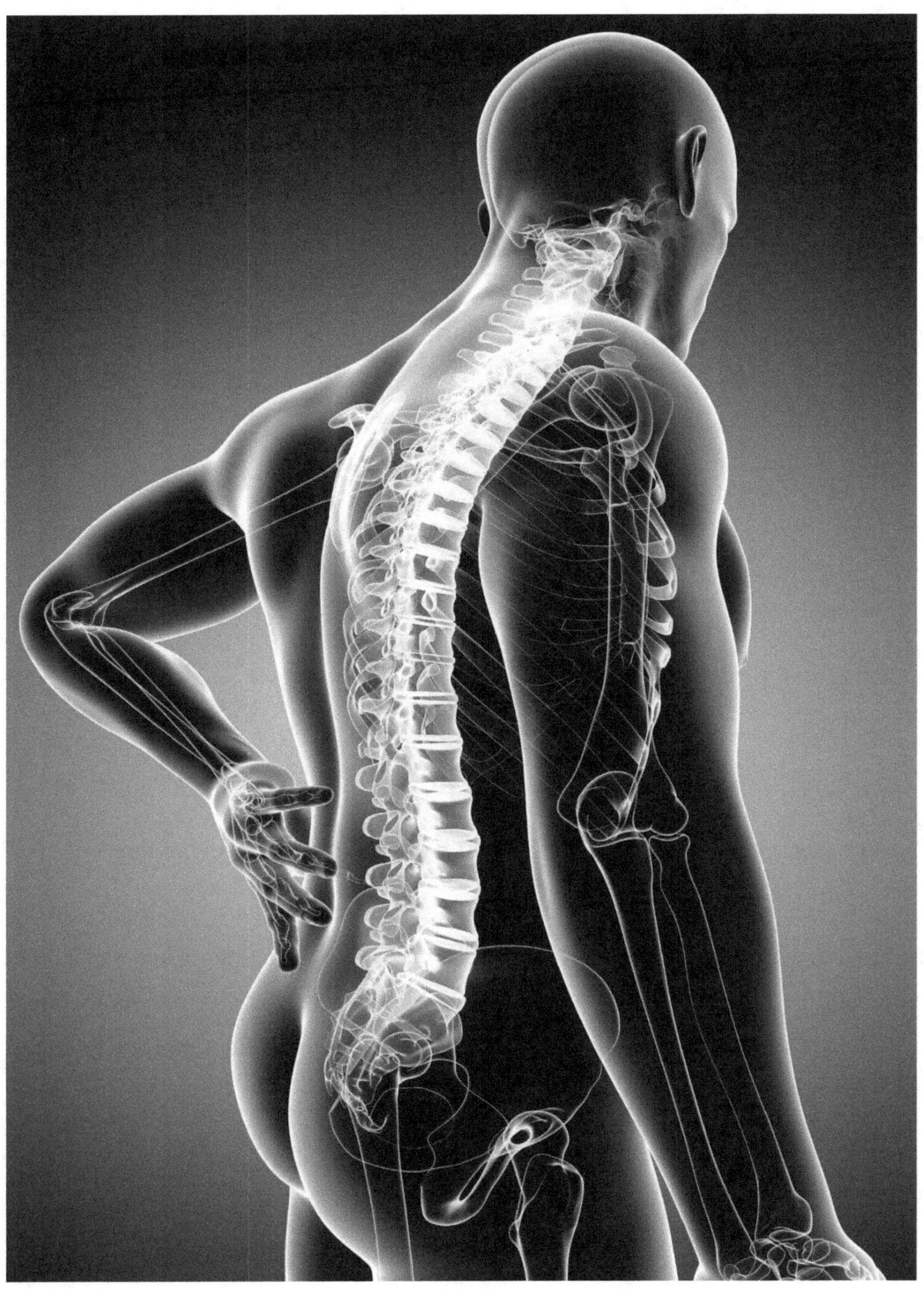

INTRODUCTION

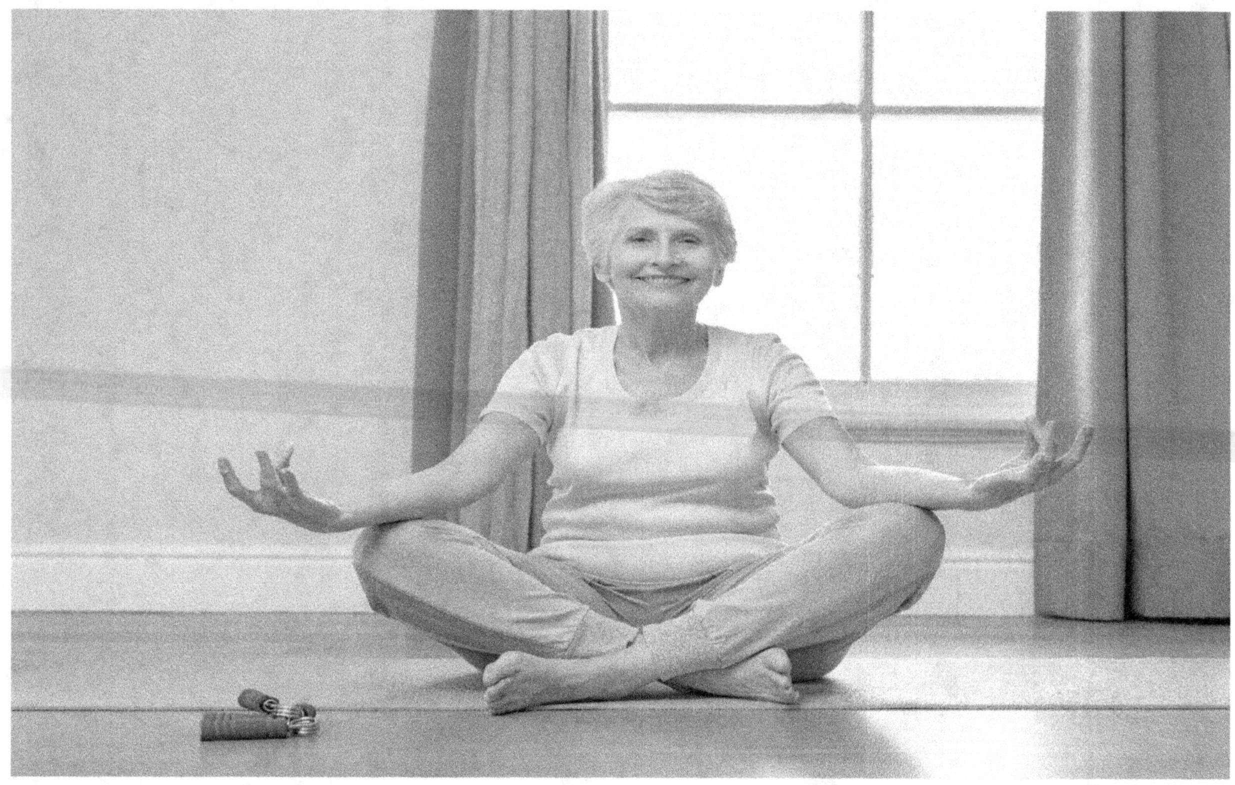

Sciatica is a widespread illness that primarily affects the elderly and millions of people globally. Sciatica can have a major negative effect on a person's quality of life. It is characterized by pain, tingling, or numbness that radiates along the sciatic nerve, which runs from the lower back down the back of each leg. This post will discuss the causes, signs, and treatment options for sciatica, with an emphasis on how exercise might help older adults with the condition.

Overview of Sciatica

Sciatica is a sign of an underlying issue, such as degenerative disc disease, spinal stenosis, or a herniated disc. It is not a separate disorder. Lower back, buttocks, and leg pain, inflammation, and discomfort can result from compression or irritation of the sciatic nerve. Prolonged sitting, standing, or moving may exacerbate this discomfort, which can range in intensity from mild to severe.

Importance of Exercise for Sciatica Relief

To manage and reduce the symptoms of sciatica, exercise is essential. The following are the top five reasons that exercise is crucial for relieving sciatica:

1. Strengthens Muscles: Consistent exercise helps the muscles that surround the spine become more robust, which improves the affected area's stability and support.

2. Enhances Flexibility: Mobility exercises and stretches make muscles and joints more flexible, which lessens stiffness and increases range of motion.

3. Encourages Better Posture: Exercise encourages the spine to be properly aligned, which lessens the pressure on the sciatic nerve and eases the discomfort brought on by bad posture.

4. Improves Circulation: Exercise increases blood flow to the injured area, supplying vital nutrients and oxygen to the injured tissues and encouraging their recovery.

5. Enhances Endorphin Release: Exercise triggers the body's natural painkillers, endorphins, to be released, which reduces pain and elevates mood.

Benefits of Exercise for Seniors

Exercise has many advantages for elders beyond just relieving sciatica. These are the top five advantages of exercise for aging bodies:

1. Enhances Balance and Coordination: Exercise lowers the chance of falls and injuries by preserving balance and coordination.

2. Preserve Bone Density: By lowering the risk of osteoporosis and fractures, weight-bearing activities help maintain bone density.

3. Preserves Muscle Mass: Seniors can keep their freedom and mobility by engaging in strength training exercises, which assist preserve muscle mass, strength, and function.

4. Improves Joint Flexibility: As we age, stiffness and discomfort are reduced by increasing joint mobility with stretches and flexibility exercises.

5. Enhances Mental Health: Research indicates that physical activity lowers stress, anxiety, and depressive symptoms, which in turn enhances mental health and general well-being.

The exercises and methods that seniors can use to properly manage their sciatica and enhance their general well-being will be covered in more detail in the sections that follow.

UNDERSTANDING SCIATICA

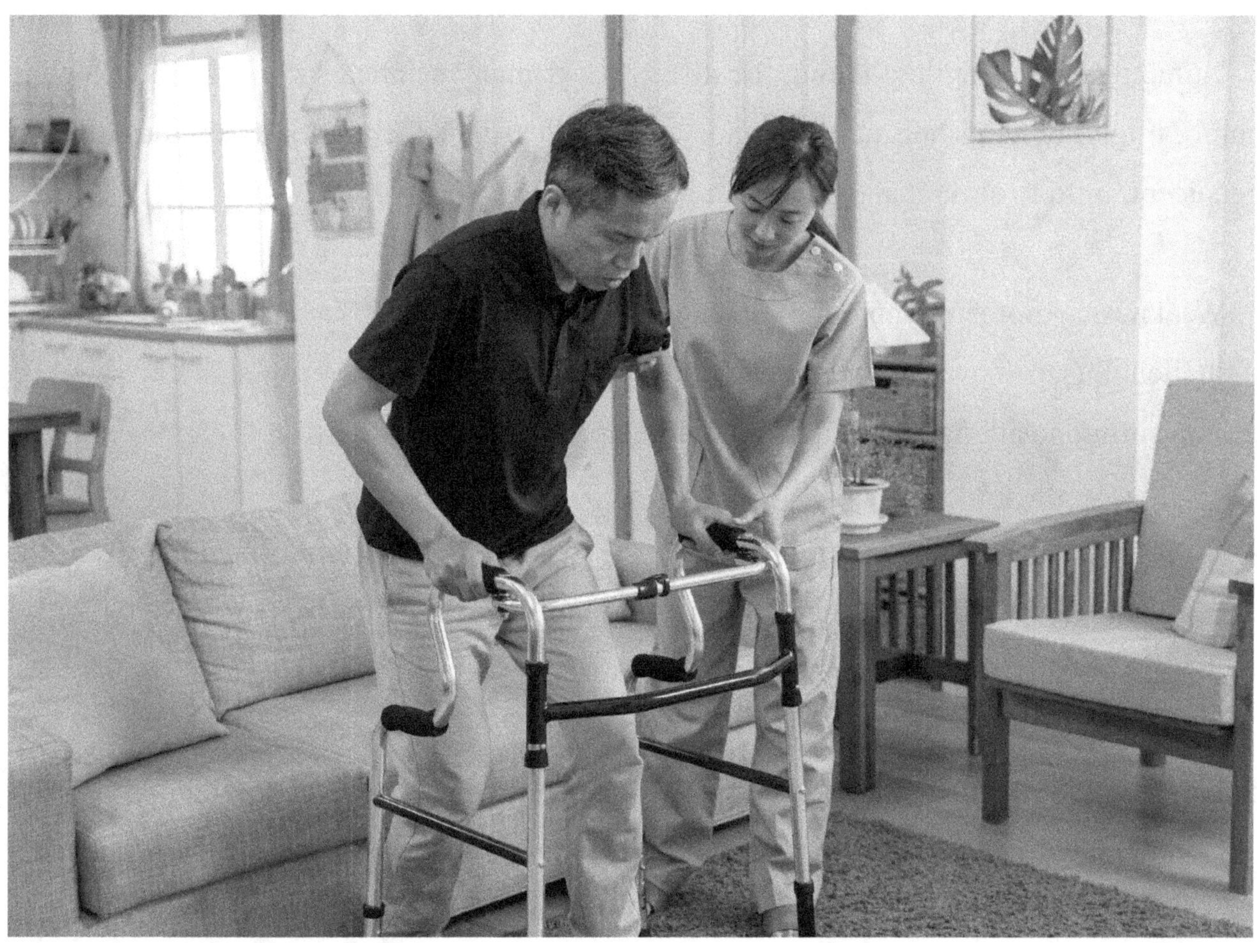

Definition and Symptoms

The hallmark of sciatica is pain that travels down each leg, passing through the hips, buttocks, and lower back before returning to the lower back. The longest nerve in the body supplies feeling to your thighs, legs, and feet as well as controlling the muscles in your lower legs.

1. Pain: The primary sign of sciatica is pain that travels down one leg and from your lower back through your buttocks. There is a wide range of pain that might range from a slight ache to a strong burning feeling or unbearable anguish. Prolonged standing, walking, or sitting may make it worse.

2. Numbness and Tingling: Along the affected leg, many sciatica sufferers report feeling numb, tingly, or as if their nails are pins and needles. This feeling may be intermittent or persistent, mild to severe, and come and go.

3. Weakness: Another symptom of sciatica is weakness in the affected leg, which makes it challenging to move or support weight. When attempting to ascend stairs or stand up from a sitting position, this weakness could be particularly apparent.

4. Radiating Pain: Sciatica pain usually has a characteristic pattern, extending from the lower back down the calf, back of the leg, and even into the foot or toes. Sharp or stabbing pain that gets worse in specific positions or movements.

5. Worsening Symptoms: Sciatica symptoms may get worse over time, particularly if they are ignored or made worse by particular activities. The quality of your life and your everyday activities can be greatly impacted by chronic sciatica, therefore getting the right therapy is crucial.

It is essential to comprehend the meaning and signs of sciatica to properly diagnose and treat this ailment. We will examine the causes, risk factors, and diagnosis of sciatica in the ensuing sections to give you a thorough grasp of this prevalent condition.

Anatomy of the Nervous System and Spine

Understanding the fundamentals of the spine's and the nerve system's anatomy is crucial to understanding sciatica. The spinal column, which supports and shields the spinal cord, is made up of a group of joined vertebrae that make up the spine. The sciatic nerve, which emerges from the lower lumbar and sacral areas of the spine, is one of the nerves that branch out from the spinal cord. Any inflammation or compression of the sciatic nerve can cause pain, numbness, and weakness along the sciatic nerve's course, which are the typical symptoms of sciatica.

Common Reasons for Senior Sciatica

Numerous underlying disorders, many of which become more common with age, can cause sciatica. Seniors' sciatica is frequently caused by the following:

1. Herniated Disc: One of the most frequent causes of sciatica, a herniated disc happens when a spinal disc's soft, gel-like center protrudes and presses against the sciatic nerve and other surrounding nerves.

2. Spinal Stenosis: This disorder causes the spinal canal to narrow, which can compress the nerves and spinal cord and cause sciatic pain. Thickened ligaments or arthritis are two examples of degenerative changes in the spine that can lead to spinal stenosis.

3. Degenerative Disc Disease: Disc bulges, herniations, and nerve compression can result from the natural aging process of the spinal discs, which causes them to lose their flexibility and shock-absorbing capacity.

4. Spondylolisthesis: This disorder results in nerve compression and sciatic sensations when a vertebra falls out of alignment and onto the vertebra underneath it.

5. Piriformis Syndrome: Symptoms like sciatica can occasionally be brought on by irritation or compression of the sciatic nerve by the piriformis muscle, which is deep within the buttocks.

Diagnosis and Treatment Options

To determine the underlying cause of the symptoms, diagnosing sciatica usually entails a comprehensive medical history, physical examination, and imaging tests like MRIs, CT scans, or X-rays. Following a diagnosis, sciatica treatment options could involve:

1. Conservative Measures: To reduce symptoms and expedite healing, conservative measures like rest, cold or heat therapy, over-the-counter painkillers, and physical therapy may be suggested.

2. Medications: To treat the pain and discomfort brought on by sciatica, doctors may occasionally prescribe prescription pharmaceuticals such as muscle relaxants, anti-inflammatory drugs, or medications for nerve pain.

3. Injections: Temporary relief from sciatic pain and inflammation reduction can be achieved by administering corticosteroid injections directly into the afflicted area.

4. Surgery: Discectomy or laminectomy are two surgical procedures that may be considered to relieve pressure on the sciatic nerve in cases of severe sciatica that do not improve with conservative measures.

To properly manage sciatica and enhance the quality of life for seniors, it is imperative to have a thorough understanding of the anatomy, typical causes, diagnosis, and available treatments. We will look at particular stretches and methods to relieve sciatica and improve general health in the upcoming chapters.

EXERCISE AND RELIEF FROM SCIATICA

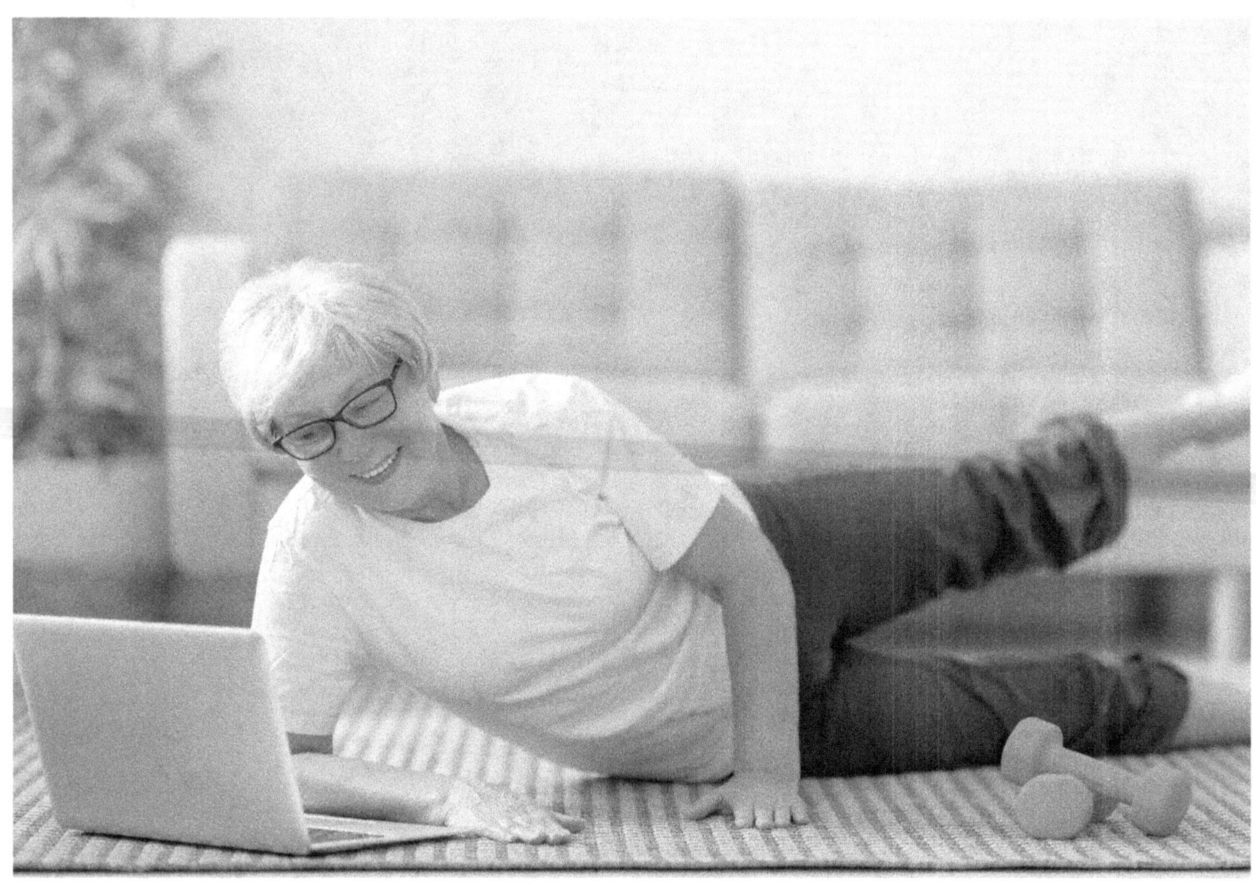

Exercise's Part in the Management of Sciatica

An essential part of managing and alleviating sciatica symptoms is exercise. During a sciatic flare-up, resting may seem like the best course of action, but being active can help reduce discomfort and avoid more episodes. Here, we look at the crucial part exercise plays in the treatment of sciatica:

1. Strengthens Supporting Muscles: Consistent exercise helps build up the back, buttocks, and core muscles that surround the spine. By making these muscles stronger, the spine is better supported and stabilized, which relieves pain by putting less strain on the sciatic nerve.

2. Enhances Flexibility and Mobility: An integral part of any program for treating sciatica is stretching and flexibility exercises. By decreasing stiffness and increasing range of motion, these exercises aid in increasing the flexibility of the muscles and joints. Improved posture and less sciatic nerve strain can be achieved by increasing flexibility, which also lowers the likelihood of further flare-ups.

3. Encourages Improved Posture and Alignment: Sciatic nerve compression and pain can be caused by poor posture and a misaligned spine. Exercise regimens emphasizing spinal alignment and posture correction can help relieve sciatic nerve irritation and lessen pain. Exercises that strengthen the back and core muscles can also help with posture and spinal stability, which lowers the chance of experiencing symptoms associated with sciatica.

4. Promotes Circulation and Healing: Exercise increases blood flow to the wounded area, supplying vital nutrients and oxygen to the injured tissues and encouraging their recovery. By releasing pressure on the sciatic nerve and reducing edema and inflammation, increased circulation can help alleviate pain.

5. Encourages General Well-Being: Research has demonstrated the many positive effects exercise has on both physical and mental health, including lowered stress levels, happier moods, and better sleep. Exercise for sciatica management not only relieves pain but also improves general health and quality of life.

You can efficiently manage sciatica symptoms, lessen discomfort, and enhance your general function and mobility by adding targeted workouts and strategies into your regimen. This chapter will cover a variety of techniques and exercises that can be used to reduce sciatic pain and encourage long-term relief in the sections that follow.

Exercise's Advantages for Sciatica Relief

There are several advantages to exercise for reducing sciatica symptoms and enhancing general health. The following are the main advantages of exercise for sciatica relief:

1. Lessens discomfort and Discomfort: By building muscle, increasing flexibility, and encouraging improved posture, regular exercise can reduce sciatic discomfort. Exercise helps lessen sciatica pain and suffering by treating the underlying causes of the problem.

2. Enhances Function and Mobility: Exercises that build strength and flexibility improve general function and mobility, which makes it simpler to carry out daily tasks with less discomfort. For those with sciatica, increased mobility improves quality of life and lowers the chance of impairment.

3. Prevents Recurrence: By strengthening supporting muscles, enhancing posture, and fostering spinal health, exercise can help stop sciatica bouts in the future. Exercise helps to lessen the likelihood of re-injury and recurrence of sciatic pain by treating muscular imbalances and deficits.

4. Encourages Healing and Recovery: Exercise increases blood flow to the wounded area, nourishing and oxygenating the injured tissues and encouraging healing. Exercise

shortens the duration of sciatica symptoms and speeds up the healing process by improving circulation and lowering inflammation.

5. Improves Mental Well-Being: Research has demonstrated that exercise improves mental health by lowering levels of stress, anxiety, and sadness. Exercise improves mood and relaxation, which improves general well-being and helps people deal with the difficulties of having sciatica.

Senior Safety Tips and Precautions

Even though exercise can reduce the symptoms of sciatica, seniors must exercise carefully to prevent aggravating their disease. The following safety advice and precautions should be remembered:

1. Speak with a Healthcare Professional: Seniors suffering from sciatica should speak with their healthcare practitioner to make sure any workout regimen is safe and suitable for their condition before beginning.

2. Start Slowly and Advance Gradually: Start with low-impact, moderate exercises and increase the length and intensity as tolerated. Steer clear of pushing through pain or overexerting yourself as this might exacerbate symptoms and cause harm.

3. Listen to Your Body: If you feel pain, discomfort, or strange symptoms throughout an activity, pay heed to your body's messages and adjust or stop the exercise. It's critical to respect your boundaries and refrain from overexerting yourself.

4. Pay Attention to Correct Form and Technique: To prevent strain and injury, perform exercises with correct form and technique. Consult a licensed physical therapist or fitness expert for advice if

you're not sure how to complete a certain exercise correctly.

5. Remain Hydrated and Take Breaks: To stay hydrated, drink lots of water before, during, and after physical activity. When you feel tired or uncomfortable, especially, take frequent pauses to relax and recuperate.

Seniors with sciatica can get the benefits of exercising for pain relief while lowering their chance of injury or aggravating their disease by heeding these safety advice and precautions.

CHAPTER 3

STRETCHING AND WARM-UP

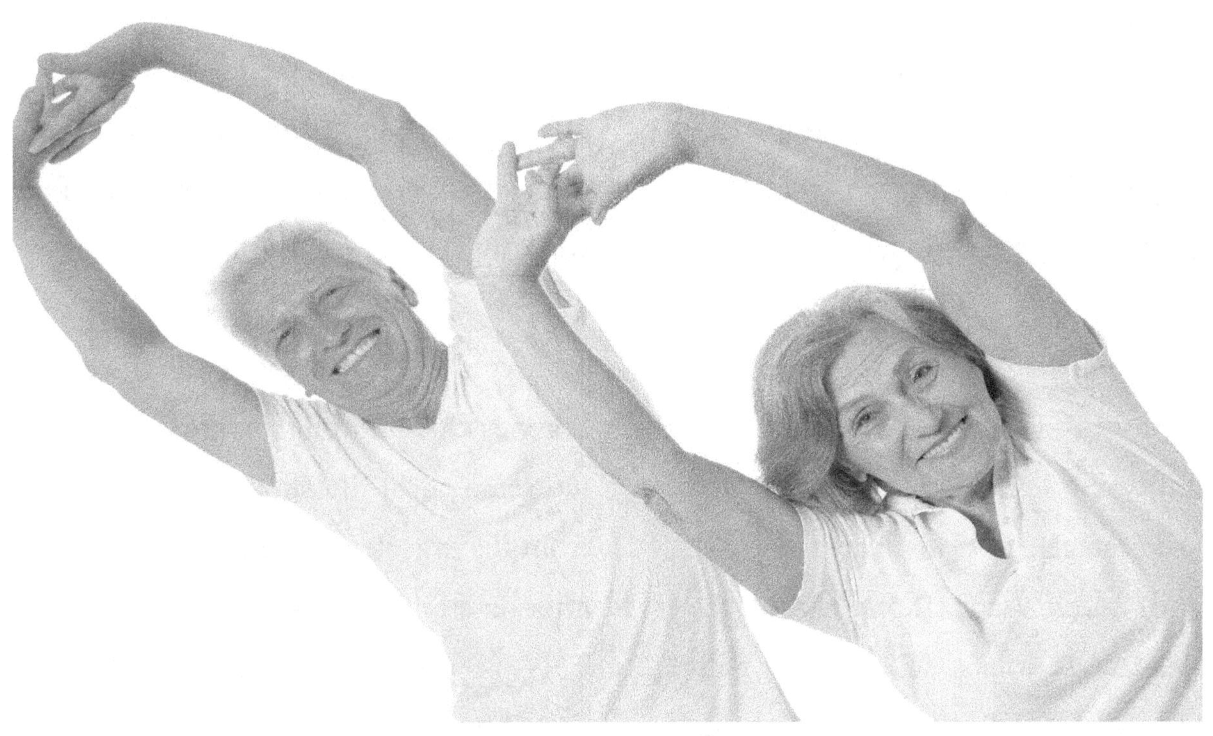

The Value of Stretching and Warming Up

Any fitness program must include a warm-up and stretching, but this is especially true for seniors who are treating sciatica. They boost blood flow to the muscles, prime the body for exercise, and enhance range of motion and flexibility. In this article, we discuss how crucial it is for seniors with sciatica to warm up and stretch:

1. Prevents Injury: A proper warm-up gets the muscles, ligaments, and tendons ready for exercise by progressively raising body temperature, heart rate, and blood flow. This lessens the possibility of getting hurt while exercising, which is crucial for those with sciatica since they

may be more vulnerable to sprains or strains of the muscles.

2. Enhances Muscle Function: Warm-up routines assist in lubricating and activating the muscles, increasing their responsiveness and efficiency. This improves muscle function, coordination, and general performance, making physical exercise for elders safer and more efficient.

3. Improves Range of Motion and Flexibility: Stretching during the warm-up stage aids in increasing the range of motion and flexibility of the muscles and joints. Exercises with correct form and technique become easier to perform as a result of the muscles becoming less tight and tense. Increased flexibility also lessens the possibility of posture issues and muscle imbalances related to sciatica.

4. Get Ready Physically and Mentally: Exercise begins with mental and physical preparation with warm-up exercises. They offer a chance to concentrate, get in the right frame of mind for the workout, and establish goals for the session. This mental readying can improve focus, motivation, and general enjoyment of the workout.

5. Accelerates Recovery and Lessens Soreness: A thorough warm-up aids in the removal of metabolic waste products from the muscles, which lessens soreness after exercise and speeds up recovery. This is especially helpful for elderly people who have sciatica since it makes it possible for them to exercise regularly without feeling too uncomfortable or worn out.

For seniors who are treating sciatica, in particular, including a comprehensive warm-up and stretching routine in your exercise regimen is crucial to optimizing the benefits of physical activity and lowering the risk of damage. We will look at particular stretches and warm-ups in the upcoming sections of this chapter to help get the body ready for safe and efficient activity.

Gentle Warm-Up Exercises for Seniors

Exercise 1: Seated Spinal Twists (Targets: Core, Lower Back)

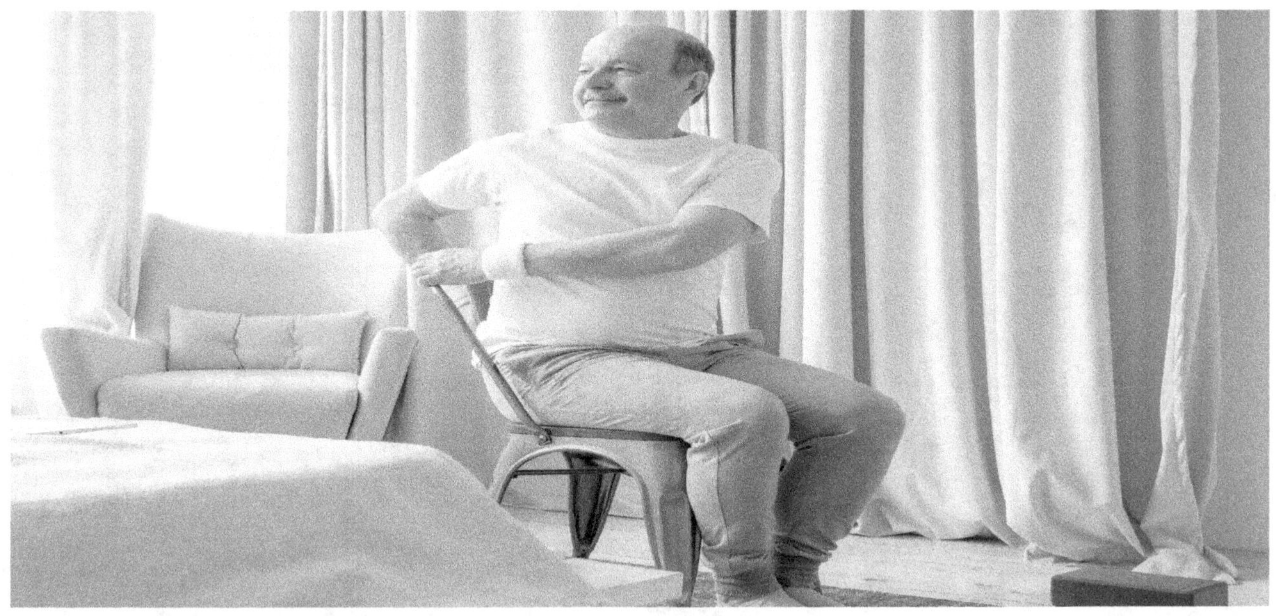

1. Place your hands on your thighs and your feet flat on the floor while you sit in a chair.

2. Breathe in and glance over your right shoulder as you slowly rotate your upper body to the right.

3. For a deeper stretch, exhale and lightly place your left hand (palm) against your right leg.

4. Take a breath and come back to the center position. Continue on the opposite side.

5. Perform five to ten reps on each side.

6. Sets: two to three

Modification: Rather than reaching across your torso, maintain your hands on your thighs for a decreased range of motion.

Avoid common errors such as hunching your shoulders, holding your breath, and twisting too forcibly.

Exercise 2: Cat-Cows Standing (Objectives: Hips, Spine)

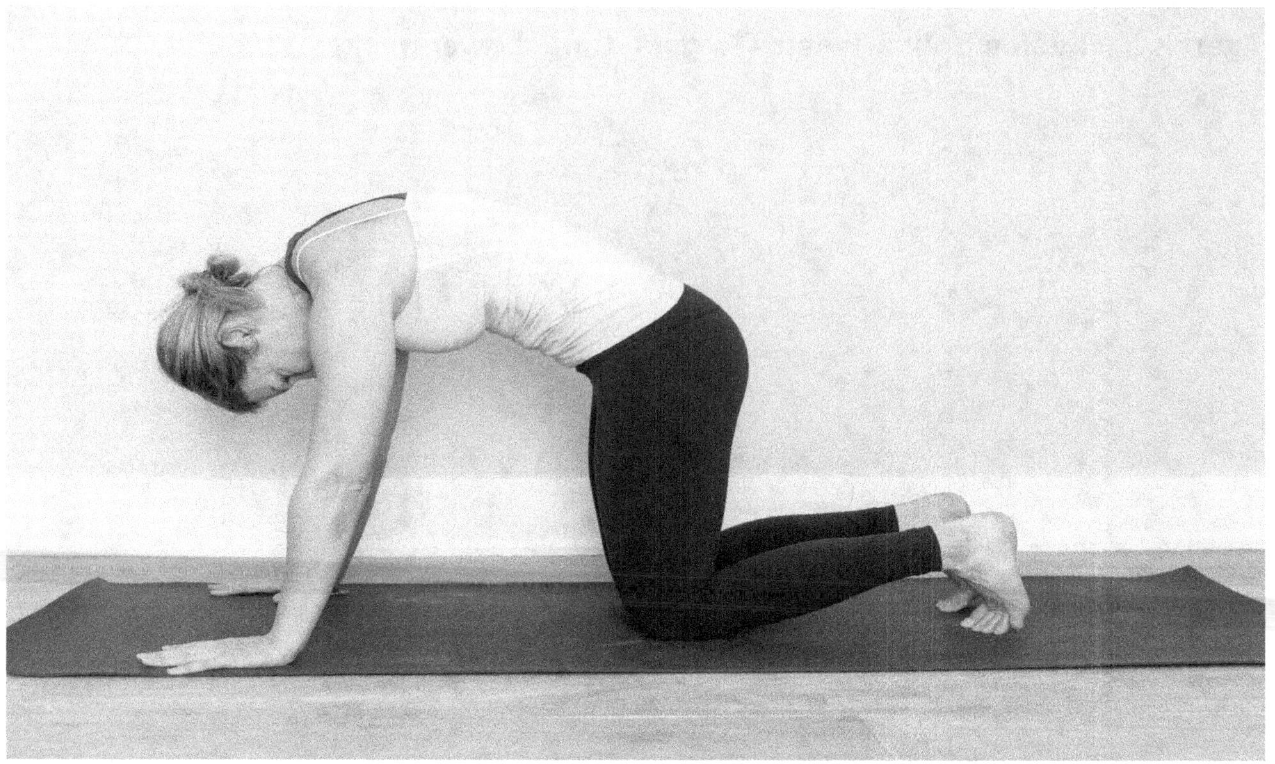

1. Pose tall, with your knees slightly bent and your feet hip-width apart.
2. Take a deep breath, arch your back, lower your head and tailbone, and pull your belly button in toward your spine to create the cow stance.
3. Exhale, round your back and assume the cat stance by tucking your chin into your chest and arching your lower back.
4. Breathe in sync with the action and repeat five to ten times.
5. Sets: 2–3.

Modification: If standing is too difficult, complete this exercise on all fours.

Avoid common blunders like straining your neck, rounding your back too much in a cat stance, and arching your back in a cow pose.

Pay close attention to how your spine moves and how each movement is in sync with your breathing.

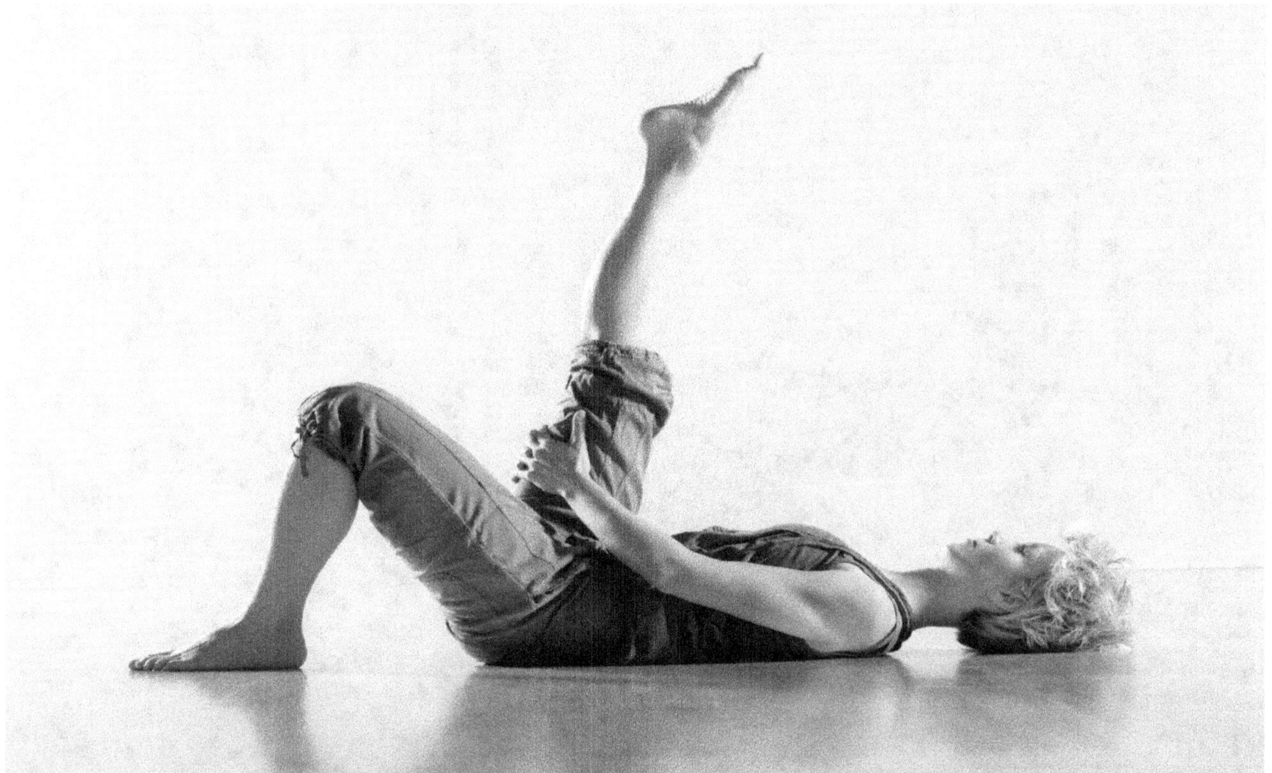

1. With your arms extended high and your feet hip-width apart, take a stance facing a wall.
2. Put your heel flat on the wall and place one foot straight back on it.
3. Lean forward from your hips, keeping your front leg straight, and reach through your heel until you feel a stretch in your hamstring.
4. Hold for a duration of 15-30 seconds. Continue on the opposite side.

Modification: If fully leaning forward is problematic, use a chair or stool for support.

Common errors to steer clear of bending forward from the shoulders rather than the hips, locking your knees, and rounding your back

For a deeper stretch, keep your front leg straight and engaged while applying strong pressure with your heel to the wall.

Exercise 4: Kneeling Glute Stretch (Targets: Glutes, Hips)

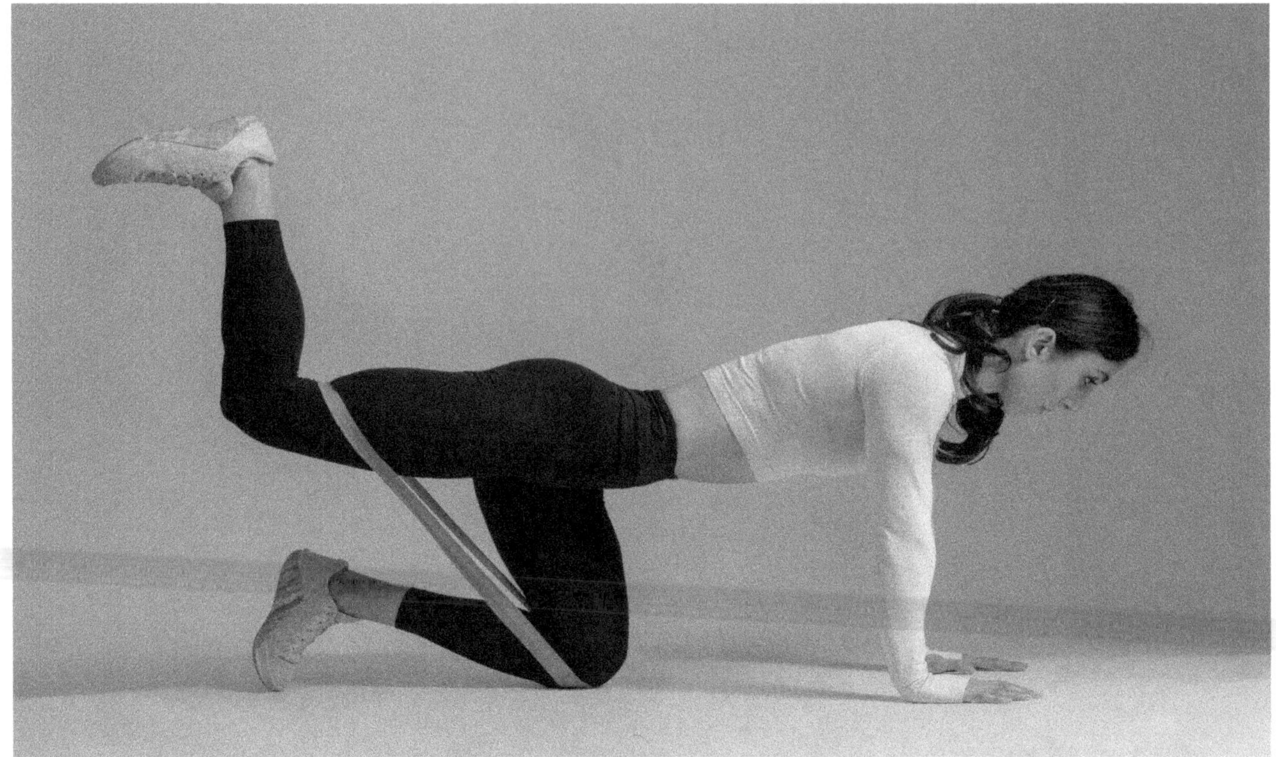

1. Place your foot flat on the floor and bend one knee while kneeling there. The other leg should be straight behind you.
2. Maintain a straight extended leg and pointed toes while you slouch slightly on your hips.
3. Maintaining a straight back, gently bend forward from your hips until you feel a stretch in your glute of the extended leg.
4. Hold for a duration of 15-30 seconds. Continue on the opposite side.

Modification: For more comfort, place a pillow or rolled-up towel beneath your knees.

Avoid common blunders including excessive forward-leaning, back arching, and unequal hips.

To maintain proper posture, keep your extended leg straight, point your toes, and contract your core.

Exercise 5: Seated Ankle Circles (Targets: Ankles, Lower Legs)

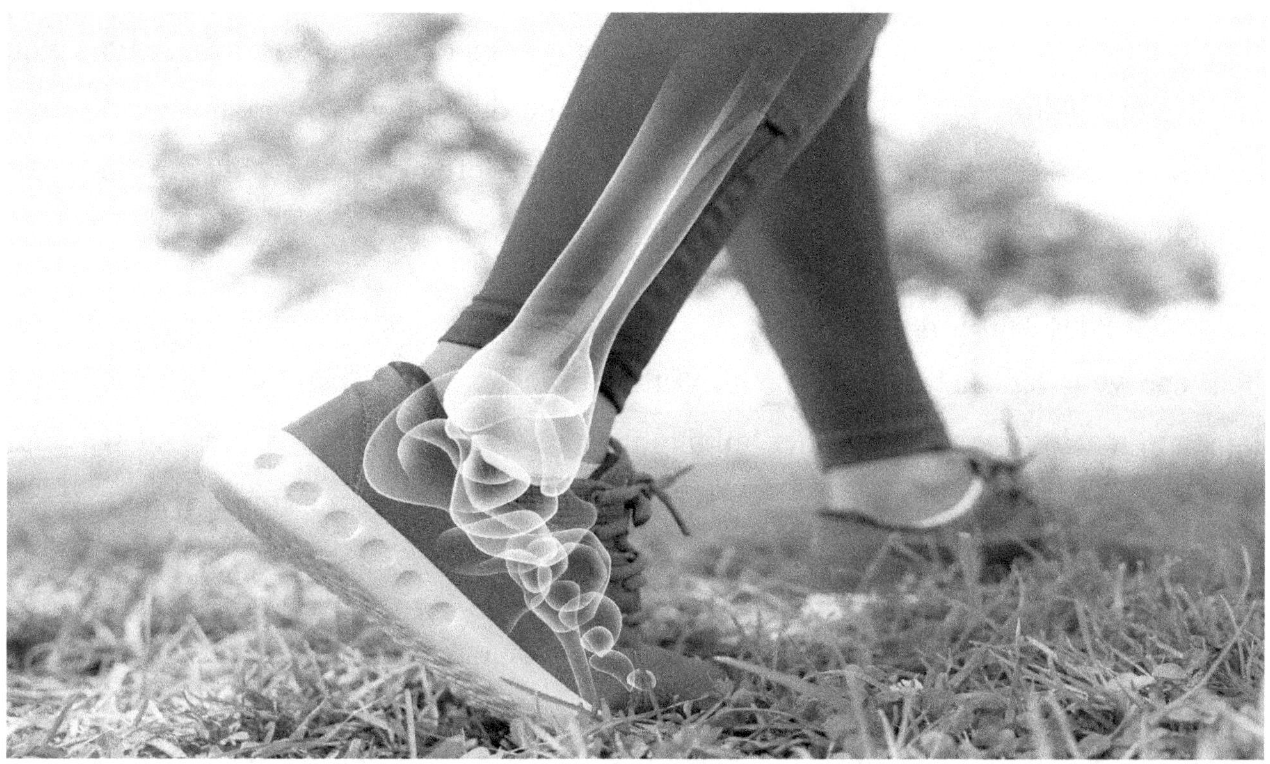

1. Place your feet flat on the ground and take a seat.
2. 5–10 slow clockwise rotations of your right ankle are performed. Continue counter-clockwise after that.
3. With your left ankle, make the same circles once again.

Modification: Try doing this exercise while lying down if sitting is too tough.

Common errors to steer clear of Using too much energy, rushing the motion, and circling your toes rather than your ankle

Steer clear of any jumping or jerking motions and concentrate on making steady, fluid circles.

Recall to pay attention to your body and cease any exercise that hurts. Throughout the warm-up, take deep breaths and concentrate on using light movements.

Stretching Technique That Work Well for Sciatica Relief

Any fitness regimen must include stretching, but it's especially important for seniors who are dealing with sciatica. Stretching relieves sciatic discomfort, lowers muscle tension, and increases flexibility. The following are some efficient stretching methods for relieving sciatica:

1. Stretch your hamstrings by sitting on the floor with one leg outstretched and the other bent and your foot flat on the ground. With your leg extended, bend forward from your hips and reach for your toes. After holding the stretch for 15 to 30 seconds, switch your legs. The hamstrings, which can become tense and worsen sciatic discomfort, are the goal of this stretch.

2. Piriformis Stretch: Lay flat on your back with your feet flat on the ground and both knees bent. After crossing one foot over the other knee, slowly bring the bent knee up to your chest until your outer hip and buttocks start to expand. After holding for 15 to 30 seconds, swap your legs. This stretch works on the piriformis muscle, which when tense or inflammatory can compress the sciatic nerve.

3. Seated Spinal Twist: Extend your legs in front of you while sitting on the floor. One knee should be bent, and the foot should be flat on the floor outside the other thigh. With the other elbow on the outside of the bent knee and a slight twist to gaze over your shoulder, rotate your torso in the direction of the bent knee. After holding for 15 to 30 seconds, swap sides. Sciatic discomfort can be relieved by stretching the buttocks and spine to alleviate tension.

4. Cat-Cow Stretch: Assume a hands-and-knee position, placing your knees behind your hips and your wrists precisely beneath your shoulders. Taking a deep breath, raise your chest toward the ceiling while arching your back (cow position). Exhale, tucking your chin into your chest, and rounding your back (cat pose). Continue doing this for eight to

ten repetitions, switching between the cat and cow stances with ease. This stretch relieves lower back strain and helps to mobilize the spine.

5. Child's Pose: Begin on your hands and knees, then sit back on your heels with your forehead resting on the floor (or a cushion) and your arms out in front of you. For 30 to 60 seconds, maintain this posture while concentrating on deep breathing and relaxation. Sciatica pain can be relieved by gradually stretching the buttocks, hips, and lower back in a child's pose.

Stretching exercises should always be done slowly and softly; bouncing or jerking could damage the muscles or make sciatica symptoms worse. For best results, hold each stretch for 15 to 30 seconds and repeat two to three times on each side.

By including these efficient stretching exercises into your daily routine, seniors who are experiencing sciatica can experience improved comfort and mobility as you help to improve flexibility, reduce muscle tension, and alleviate sciatic pain.

CHAPTER FOUR

STRENGTHENING EXERCISES

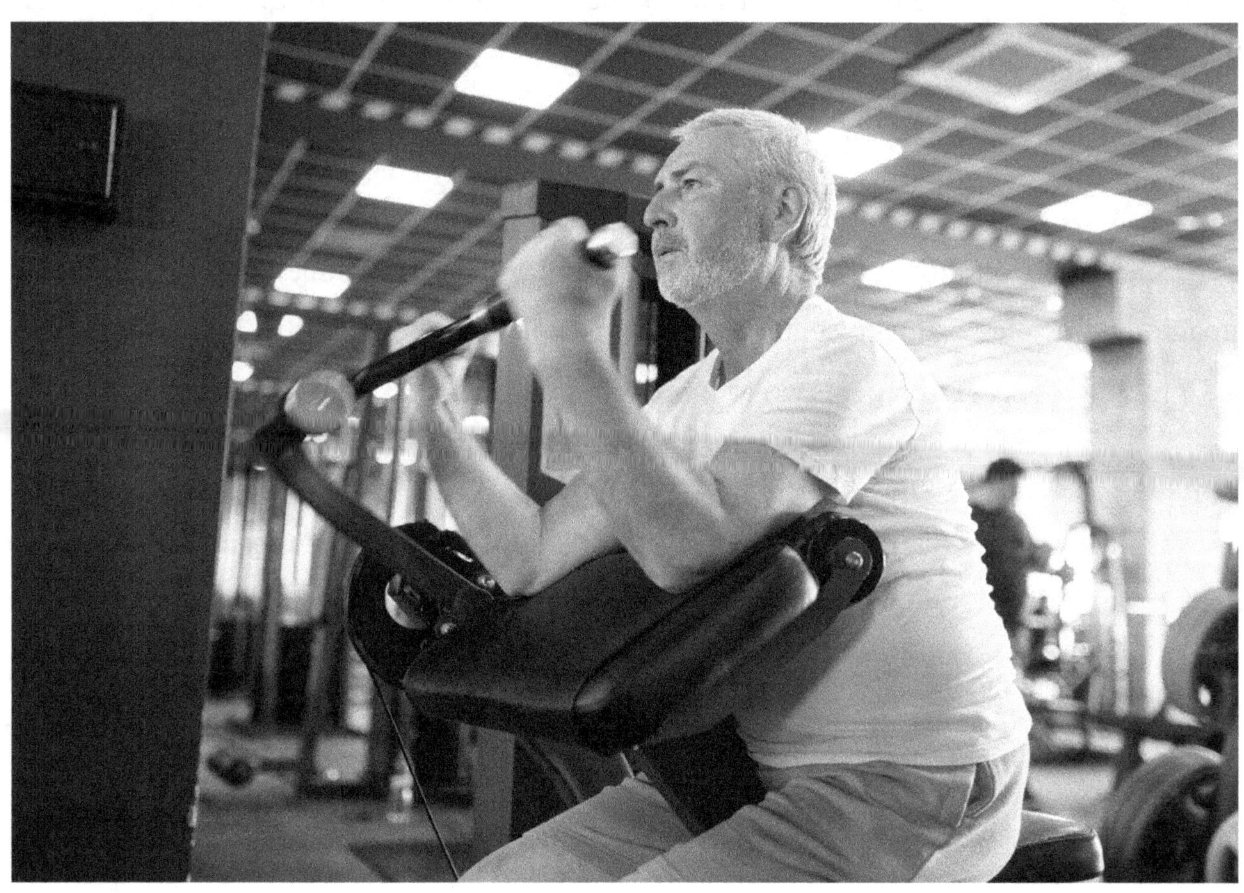

Importance of Strengthening for Sciatica Relief

An integral part of any thorough program for the alleviation of sciatica is strength training. Strengthening exercises serve to improve posture, support the spine, and relieve strain on the sciatic nerve by focusing on particular muscle groups. Here, we examine the significance of strengthening to relieve sciatica:

1. Strengthening exercises focus on the muscles that surround the spine, such as the back, buttocks, and core. This helps to stabilize the spine. By making these muscles stronger, the spine is better supported and stabilized, which lowers

the possibility of vertebral misalignment and nerve compression.

2. Enhances Posture: Improper posture can put more strain on the spine and sciatic nerve. One way to combat this is by strengthening your back and core muscles. By encouraging appropriate alignment of the spine and pelvis, strengthening exercises help to improve posture by lessening the load on the lower back and easing sciatic discomfort.

3. Lower Risk of Injury: Regular strength training is crucial for preventing injuries in people with sciatica since strong muscles are less likely to sustain an injury. By enhancing muscle endurance, coordination, and resilience, strengthening exercises help lower the risk of sprains, strains, and other musculoskeletal ailments.

4. Enhances Functional Mobility: By increasing general function and mobility, strengthening exercises help people carry out daily tasks more easily and with less discomfort. People with sciatica can move more confidently and effectively by building their muscle strength and endurance, which lessens the impact of their condition on day-to-day activities.

5. Promotes Long-Term Relief: For long-term sciatica relief, strengthening the muscles around the spine and pelvis is essential. Frequent strength training improves quality of life and provides long-lasting pain relief by addressing underlying muscular imbalances and deficits that fuel sciatic symptoms

Including strengthening activities in your regimen is crucial to controlling your sciatica symptoms and lowering your chance of recurrence. In the sections that follow, we'll look at certain strengthening exercises that focus on important muscle groups that support the spine and reduce sciatic discomfort.

Gentle Strengthening Exercises for Seniors

The following exercises, which can be performed by seniors who are active or who have restricted mobility, are aimed at strengthening the areas that are frequently impacted by sciatica pain:

Warm-up (five to ten minutes):

1. Standing Neck Rolls: Make five gentle clockwise and five gentle counterclockwise circles with your head.
2. Arm Circles: Five times in each direction, make little circles with your arms moving forward and backward.
3. Ankle Circles: Make ten rotations of your ankles in each direction, clockwise and counterclockwise.

Exercise

For Active Seniors:

Exercise 1. Glute Bridges (Glutes, Hamstrings as Targets):

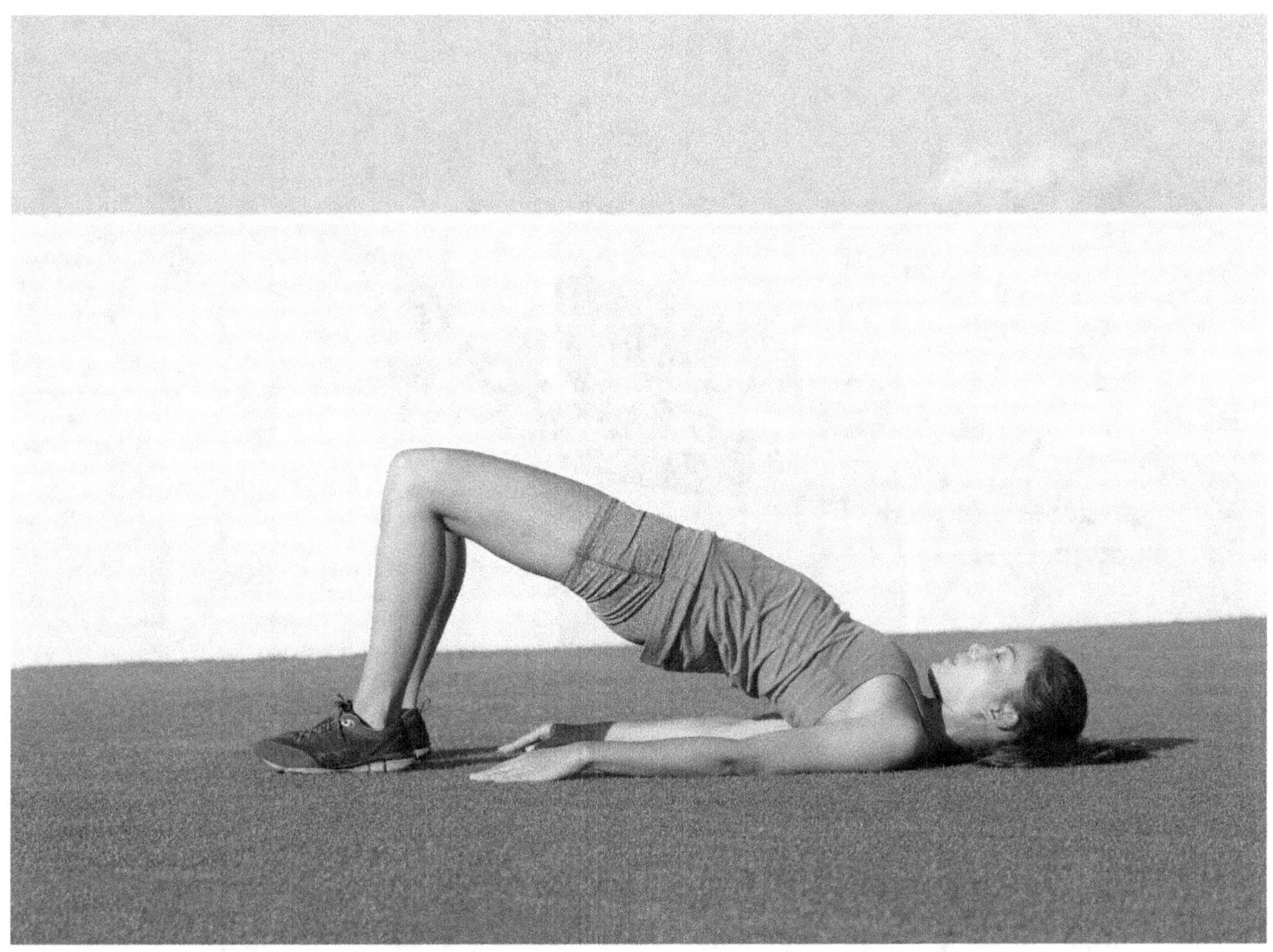

1. With your feet flat on the ground and your knees bent, lie on your back.
2. Squeeze your glutes as you raise your hips off the ground. Hold for five seconds, then gently let go.

Modification: For an extra challenge, try performing with just one leg outstretched at a time.

Sets/Reps: Three sets of ten to fifteen reps.

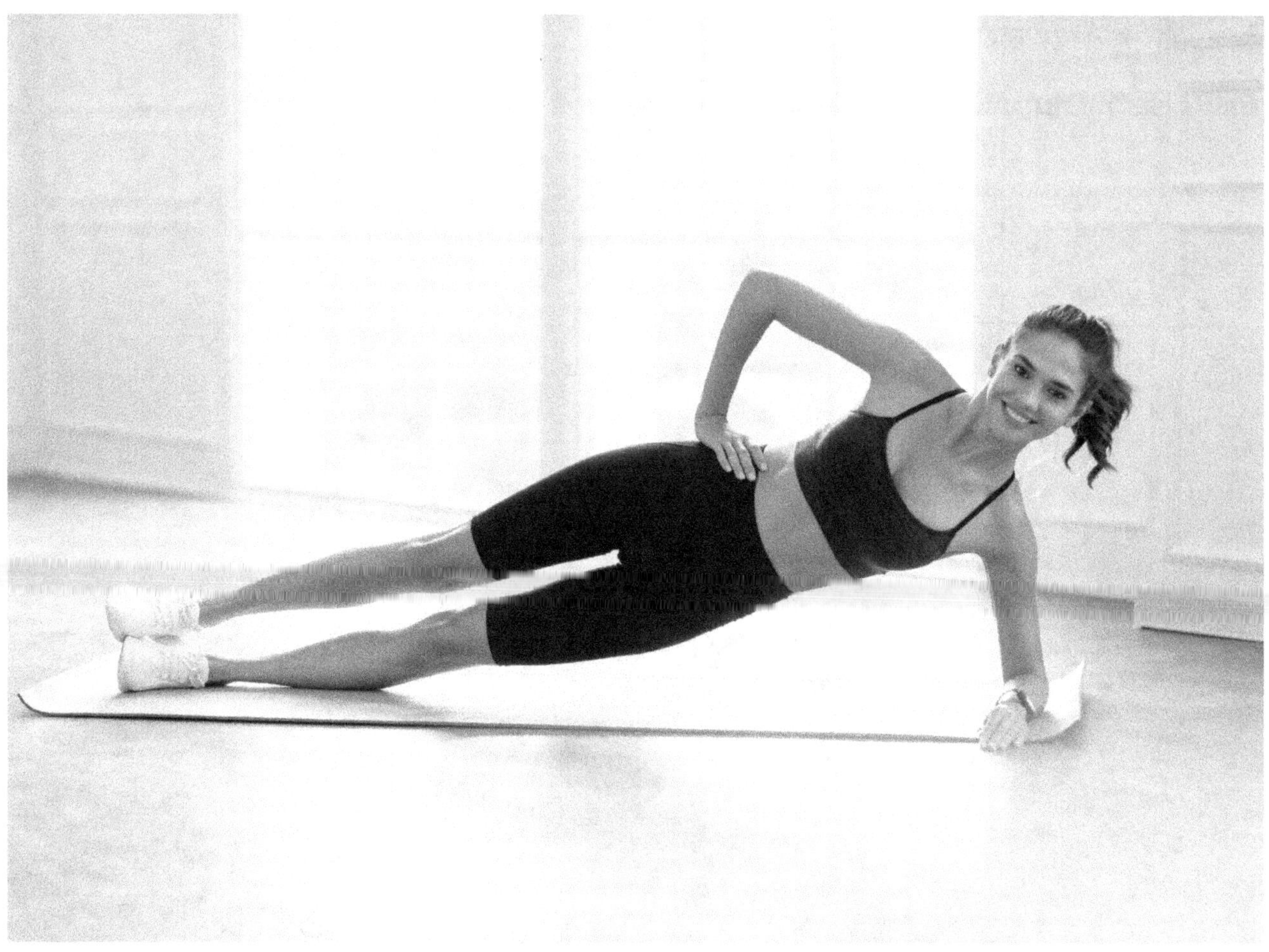

1. With your forearm flat on the floor and your elbow just under your shoulder, lie on your side.

2. Raise your hips off the floor so that your head and heels are in a straight line.

3. After holding for ten to thirty seconds, swap sides.

4. Adjustment: To ease the strain, drop your knees to the floor.

5. Sets/Reps: 3 sets, each lasting 10–30 seconds.

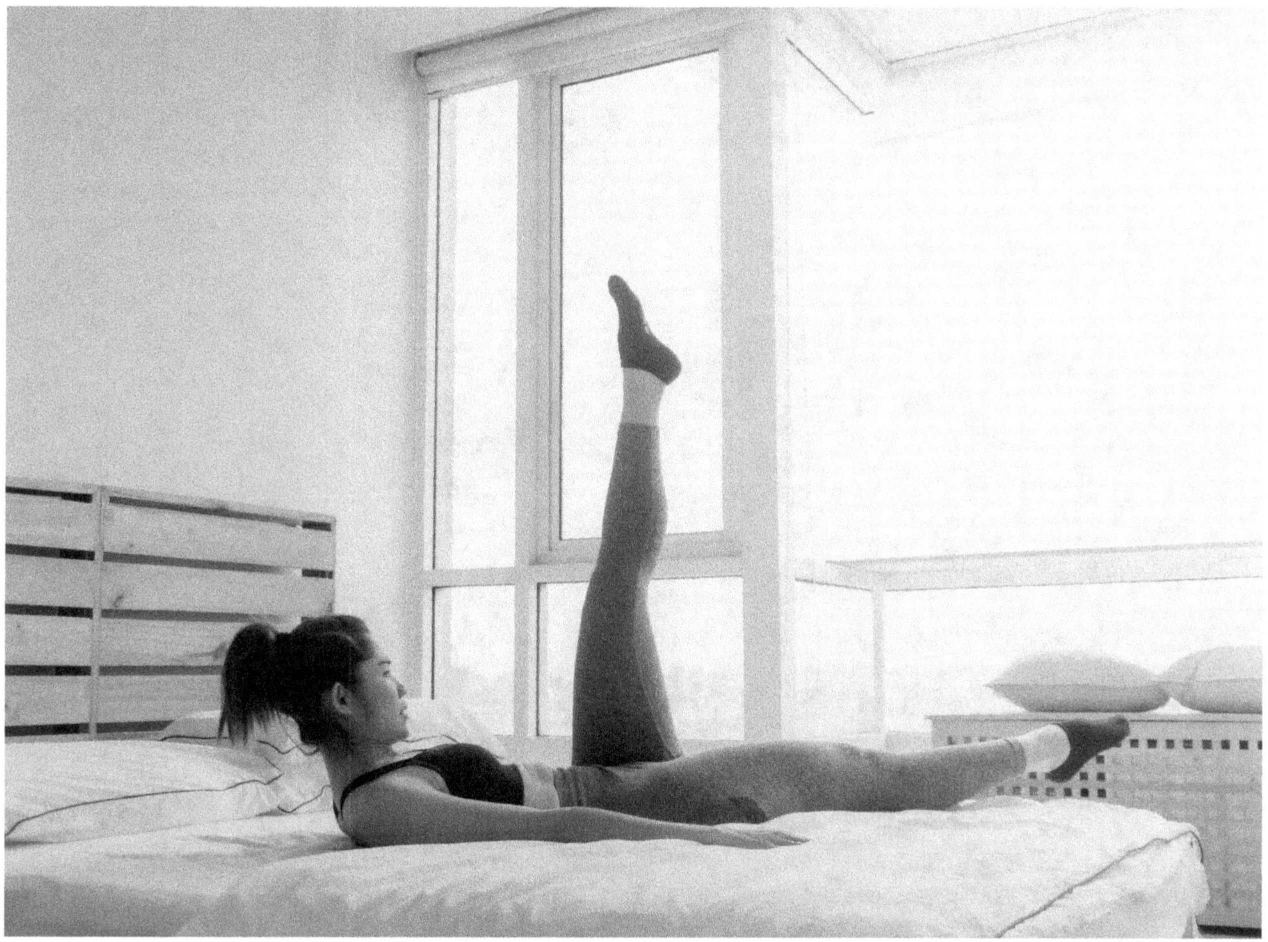

1. Extend your legs while lying on your back.

2. Lift one leg straight up toward the ceiling and slowly lower it until it is at a comfortable height.

3. Gently lower, then switch to the other leg.

Modification: If lifting a straight leg is difficult, keep your knee slightly bent.

Sets/Reps: Three sets of ten to fifteen reps for each leg.

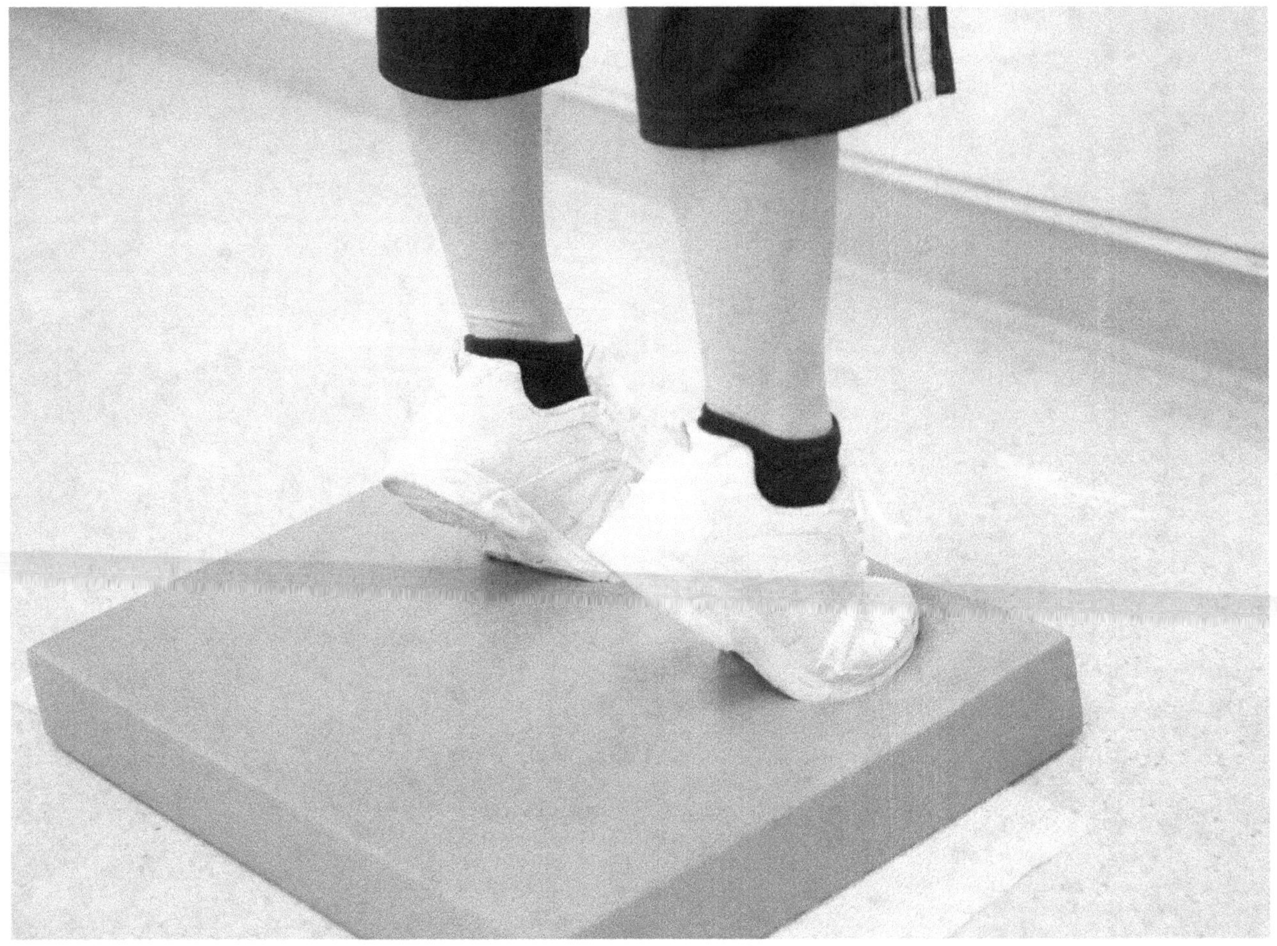

1. Put your feet hip-width apart and stand tall.
2. Squeeze your calves and lift your heels off the floor. Hold for three seconds, then gently let go.

Modification: If you need balance, grab onto a chair or wall.

Sets/Reps: Three sets of fifteen to twenty reps.

Exercise 1. Seated Knee Extensions (Targets: Quads)

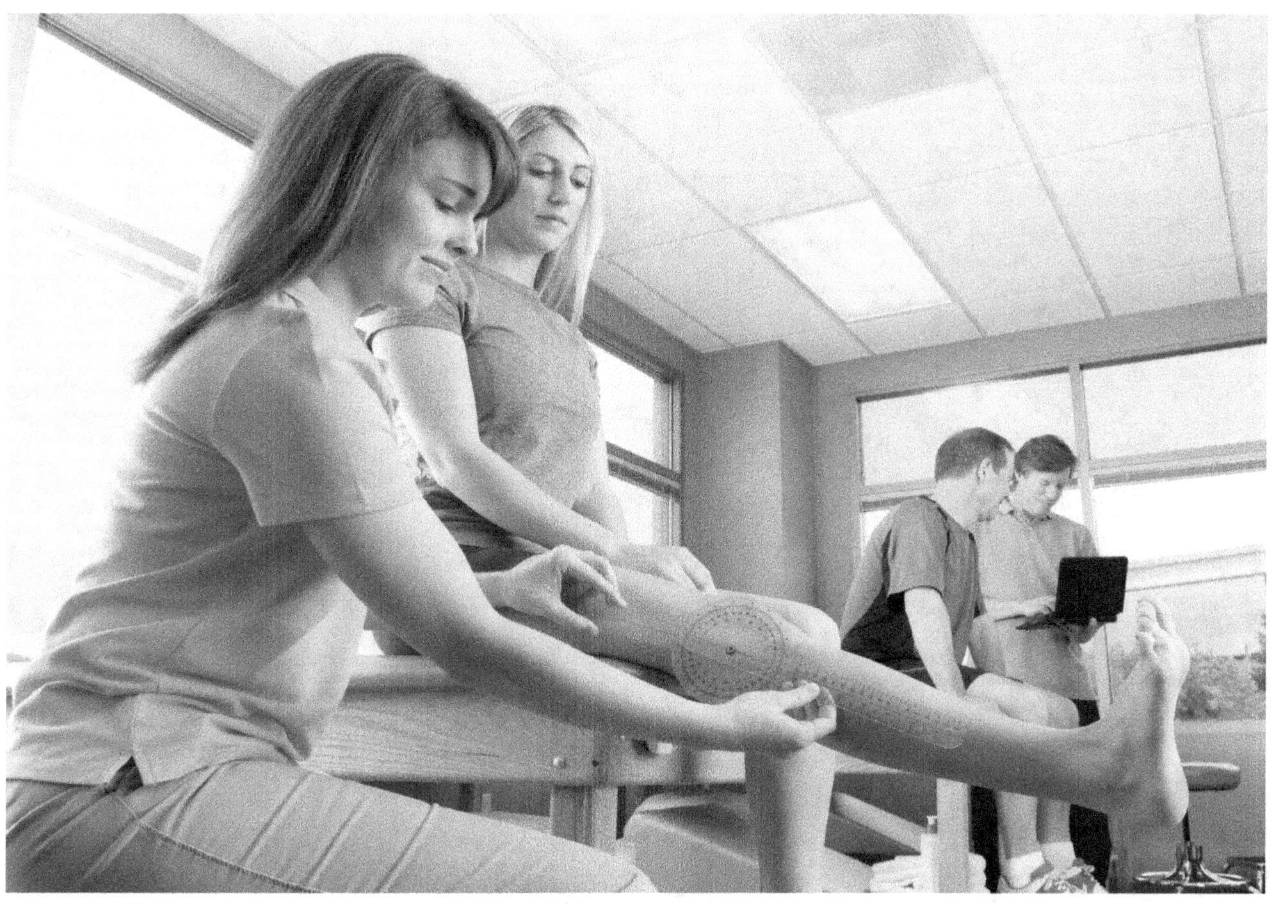

1. Place your feet flat on the ground and take a seat.

2. Stretch one leg straight in front of you and keep it there for five seconds.

3. Lower yourself gently, then switch to the other leg.

Modification: To help raise your leg, wrap a towel or strap around your ankle.

Sets/Reps: Three sets, ten reps for each leg.

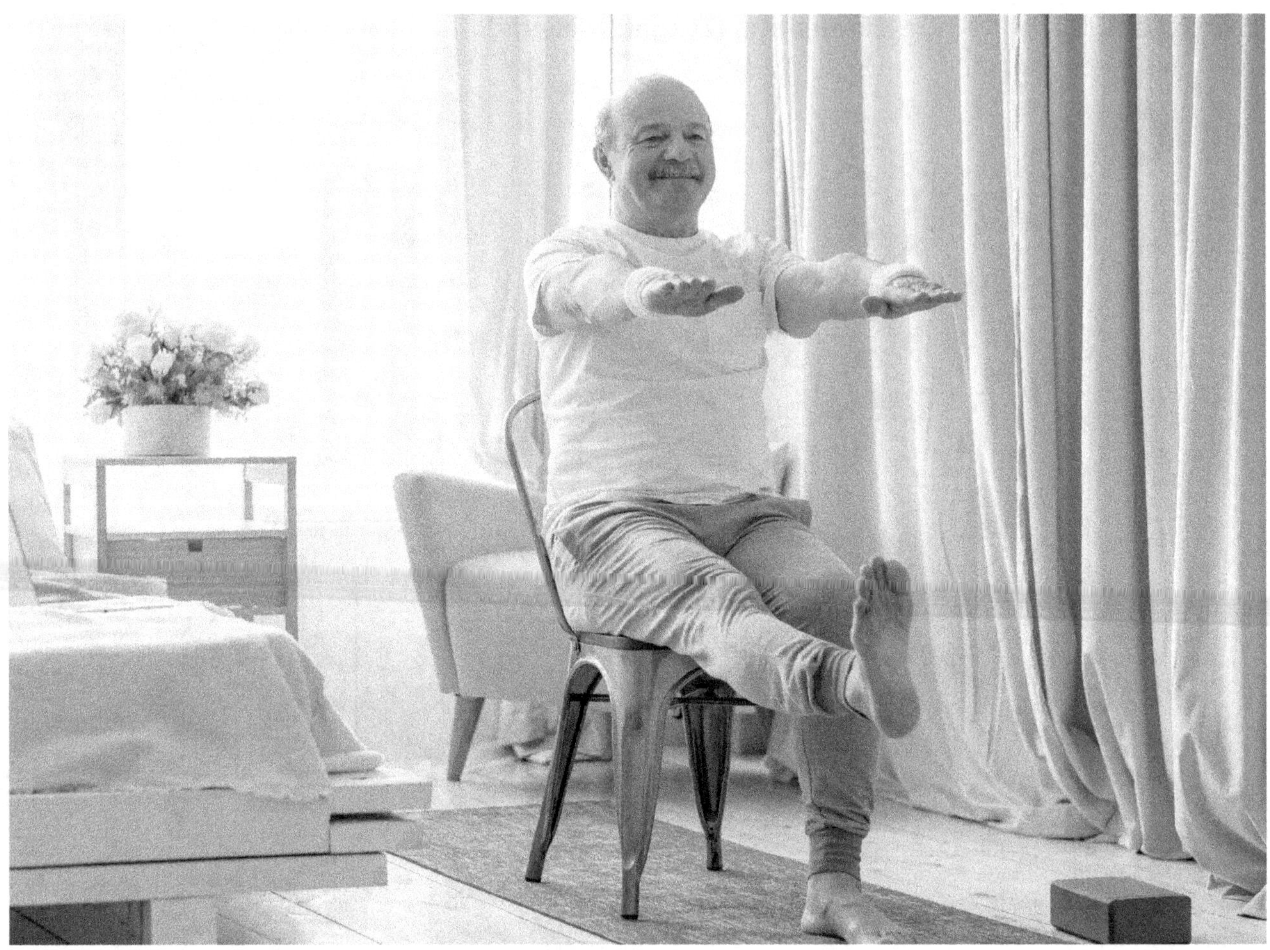

1. Sit in a chair with knees bent and feet flat on the floor.

2. Raise one knee as far as it is comfortable, hold it for five seconds, and then bring it back down.

3. Continue with the opposite leg.

Modification: For stability, keep your hands on the chair's seat.

Sets/Reps: Three sets, ten reps for each leg.

Exercise 3. Wall Leg Slides (Hamstrings and Glutes as Targets):

1. Place your hands flat on the wall in front of you for support.
2. Maintaining a straight leg, slowly move one heel up the wall as high as is comfortable.
3. Slowly descend again, then switch to the other leg.

Modification: If standing is difficult for you, complete this exercise while seated on a chair.

Sets/Reps: Three sets, ten reps for each leg.

Exercise 4. Ankle Pumps (Calves as the Target)

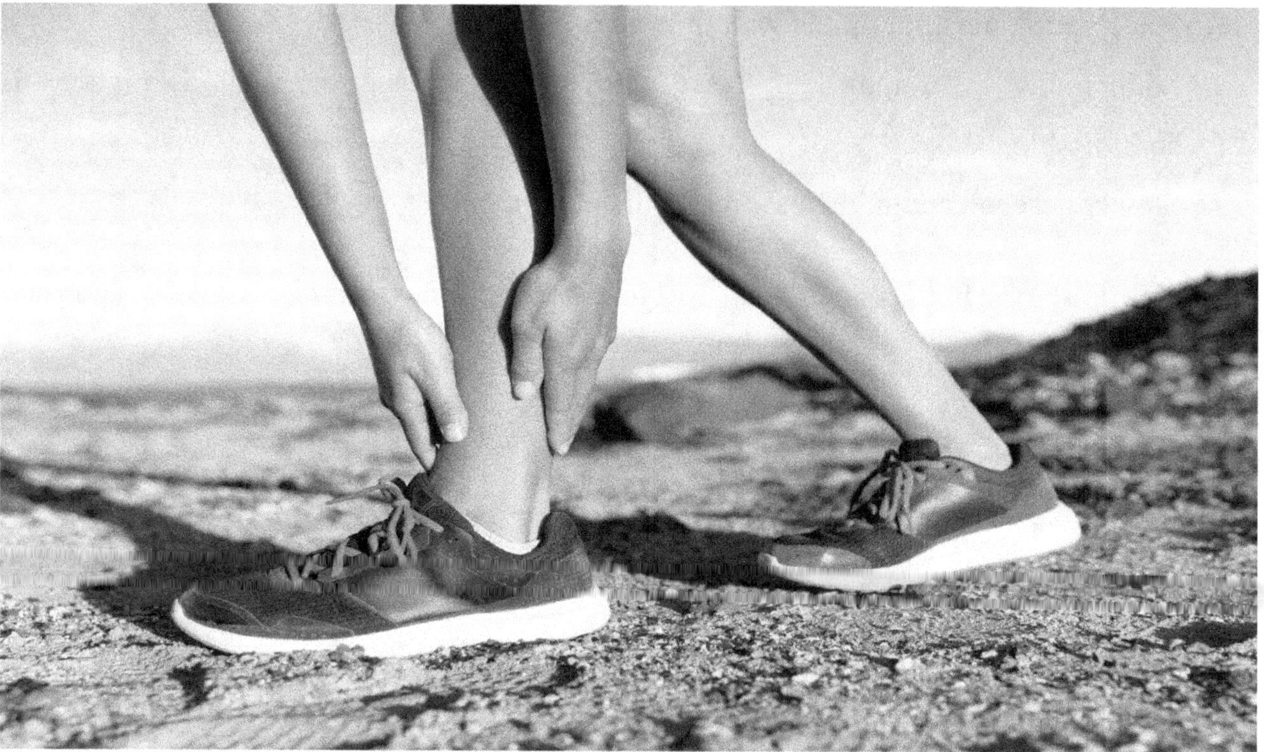

1. Place your feet flat on the ground and take a seat.

2. Take a five-second hold while pointing your toes, then let go.

3. For five seconds, curl your toes in your direction.

4. Ten times over, repeat.

5. 5-to 10-minute cool-down

Stretching exercises for the main muscle groups.

Practice deep breathing.

Increase the number of repetitions and sets gradually at first.

Pay attention to your body's signals and cease any workout that hurts.

Exercises to Strengthen Your Core and Support Your Spine

To stabilize the spine and pelvis, provide a strong base for movement, and lessen the strain on the lower back, the core muscles are essential. For those who suffer from sciatica, strengthening their core muscles is especially crucial because it can lessen discomfort and relieve pressure on the sciatic nerve. To support the spine, try these exercises to strengthen the core:

1. Plank: Begin in the push-up position, placing your hands squarely beneath your shoulders and aligning your head, shoulders, and heels in a straight line. Hold this posture for 20 to 30 seconds, or for as long as you can with proper form, by contracting your core muscles. Increase the length gradually as your strength increases.

2. Bridge: Place your feet flat on the floor and bend your knees while lying on your back. With your palms facing down, place your arms by your sides. After your hips are raised off the ground and your body is in a straight line from your shoulders to your knees, contract your core and glutes. Reposition after ten to fifteen seconds of holding. Do eight to ten repetitions.

3. Dead Bug: Arrange yourself on your back, arms outstretched toward the ceiling, knees bent 90 degrees. Press your lower back into the floor by using your core muscles. As you extend the other leg and slowly lower one arm overhead, maintain your lower back pressed into the floor. Go back to the beginning and repeat the process on the opposite side. For eight to ten repetitions, continue switching sides.

4. Bird Dog: Begin on all fours, placing your knees behind your hips and your wrists squarely beneath your shoulders. To keep your spine stable, contract your core muscles. While keeping your body in a straight line from your fingertips to your toes, extend one arm forward and the other leg back. After a brief period of holding, switch sides and go back to the

starting position. On each side, perform 8–10 repetitions.

5. Russian Twist: While sitting on the ground, bend your knees and place your feet flat on the ground. Keep your back straight and your core active as you gently lean back. Hold a weight or medicine ball in front of you, or clasp your hands together. Bring your hands or your weight towards the floor next to you as you turn your torso to one side. Go back to the center and do the opposite side. For eight to ten repetitions on each side, keep switching sides.

To support the spine, enhance posture, and lessen pressure on the sciatic nerve, include these exercises for strengthening the core into your routine. As your strength increases, start with a few repetitions and progressively increase the intensity and duration.

CHAPTER FIVE

EXERCISES FOR FLEXIBILITY AND MOBILITY

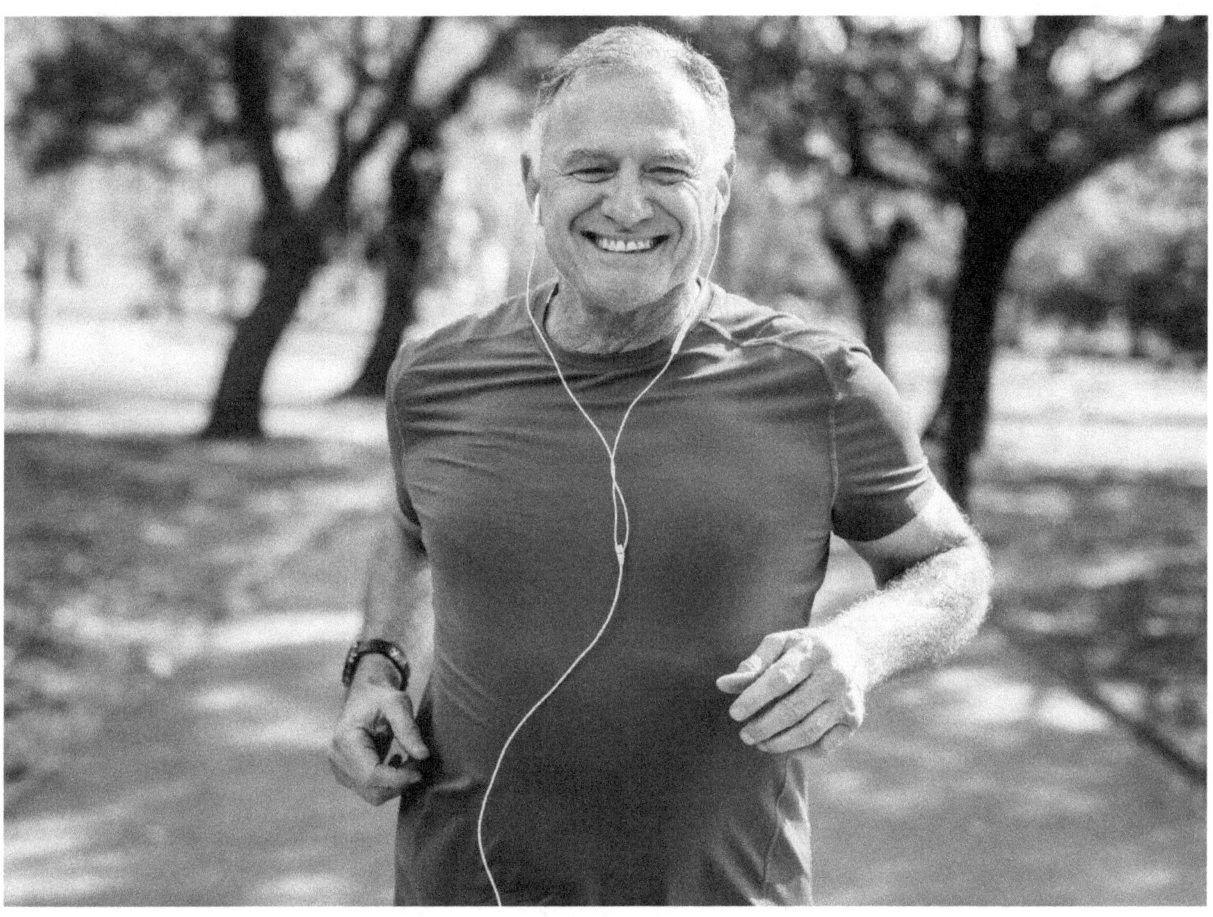

Increasing Flexibility to Reduce Sciatica

Having mobility and flexibility is crucial for controlling sciatica, especially in older adults. Pain along the sciatic nerve is the hallmark of sciatica, which can be made worse by tense muscles and restricted range of motion. For this reason, it's essential to include flexibility exercises in a thorough sciatica cure program to enhance comfort, mobility, and general well-being.

Targeted exercise regimens that improve flexibility can soothe tense muscles, lessen stiffness, and expand joint range of motion. Seniors can lessen sciatica agony and relieve pressure on the sciatic nerve by stretching tight muscles and increasing their flexibility. Furthermore, increased flexibility promotes better posture, spinal alignment, and general function, all of which help to reduce sciatic pain over the long run.

Stretching the muscles around the spine, hips, and legs gently is the main goal of flexibility exercises for sciatica relief. These exercises relieve sciatic pain and discomfort by promoting relaxation, increasing circulation, and releasing muscle tension. Seniors' quality of life can be enhanced and their sciatica more effectively managed by incorporating flexibility exercises into their regular regimen.

Mobility Exercises To Reduce Stiffness and Pain

Exercise 1. Spinal Twists While Seated (Core, Lower Back)

1. With your hands resting on your thighs and your feet flat on the floor, take a seat in a chair.
2. Take a breath, glance over your right shoulder, and slowly rotate your upper body to the right as far as it feels comfortable without straining.
3. For a deeper stretch, exhale and softly place your left hand (palm) against your right thigh while maintaining a relaxed posture and engaged core.
4. Breathe in and slowly come back to the center position. Continue on the opposite side.
5. Perform 5 to 10 reps on each side.

Modification: Restrict your range of motion by keeping your hands on your thighs rather than extending them across your body.

Exercise 2. Cat-Cow (Hip and Spine as Targets)

1. With your hands shoulder-width apart and your knees hip-width apart, begin on all fours. Maintain a straight spine and a long neck.
2. Take a deep breath, arch your back, lower your belly to the floor, and gaze upwards, assuming the cow stance.
3. In a cat stance, release your breath, turn your back, tuck your chin into your chest, and pull your belly button toward your spine.
4. Pay attention to synchronizing your breathing with every motion: take a breath as you arch, and release it as you circle.
5. Repeat 5–10 times in a smooth, continuous motion.

Modification: If you have trouble getting down on all fours, you can also try this exercise on your hands and knees while kneeling on a folded towel or cushion.

Exercise 3. Knee Hugs: Lower Back and Hips as Targets

1. With your feet flat on the ground and your knees bent, lie on your back.
2. Breathe deeply while putting your hands around one knee and hugging it gently to your chest.
3. Hold for ten to fifteen seconds, paying attention to any hip and lower back pain.
4. Lower the knee gradually, then switch to the opposite side.
5. Perform 5–10 rounds on each side.

Modification: Should you find it painful to hug your knee to your chest, try holding it halfway up or seeking support from a strap or cloth.

Exercise 4. Ankle Circles (Lower Legs and Ankles as Targets)

1. Position your feet hip-width apart and take a seat or stand.

2. 5–10 slow clockwise rotations of your right ankle should be followed by a counterclockwise rotation.

3. With your left ankle, make the same circles once again.

4. Keep your movements deliberate and fluid; steer clear of jerking or bouncing.

Modification: If you have trouble standing, do this exercise while seated or lying down.

Exercise 5. Pigeon Pose: (Hip and glute targets)

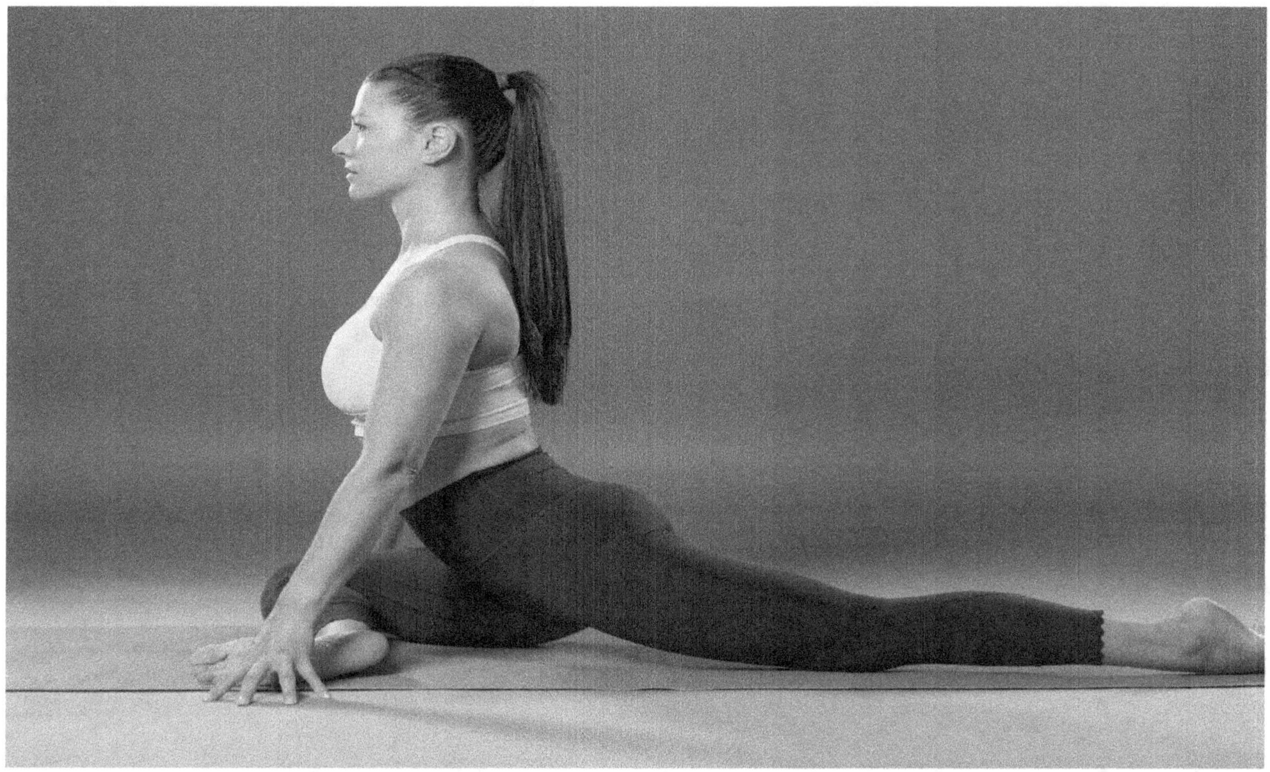

1. With your hands shoulder-width apart and your knees hip-width apart, begin on all fours.

2. With your right shin parallel to the left border of the mat, bring your right knee forward and place it between your hands. Straighten your left leg and place it back on your toes or the top of your foot.

3. Sit up straight, squaring your hips and using your core.

4. Take a deep breath, hold it for 30 to 60 seconds, and pay attention to any feelings in your glutes and hips.

5. Continue on the opposite side.

Modification: If you find it painful to move your knee forward, support your shin with a block or pillow.

This pose can also be executed as a figure-four, with both knees bent and stacked.

Pay attention to your body's signals and cease any workout that hurts.

Adjust these workouts to suit your unique fitness level and limits as necessary.

Be sure to speak with your physician or physical therapist before beginning a new fitness regimen.

Tai Chi and Gentle Yoga for Seniors with Sciatica

Tai Chi and gentle yoga are age-old techniques with many advantages for elderly people with sciatica. These mindful movement exercises are perfect for those with sciatica pain since they include mild stretching, strengthening, and relaxing approaches. This chapter will look at the benefits of mild yoga and Tai Chi for seniors experiencing sciatica and wanting to feel better overall.

Mild Yoga for the Relief of Sciatica

Yoga is a holistic discipline that enhances flexibility, balance, and calmness through the use of physical postures, breathing exercises, and meditation. The emphasis of gentle yoga is on slow, deliberate movements that can be modified to meet the needs and limits of each individual. Gentle yoga can help seniors with sciatica feel less stressed, more flexible, and less in pain.

The advantages of gentle yoga for elderly people with sciatica

1. Stretching and Strengthening: To improve posture and spinal alignment, do mild yoga poses that target the muscles that surround the spine and pelvis. Yoga can help relieve sciatic nerve irritation and lessen discomfort by treating muscular imbalances and limitations.

2. Increased Range of Motion and Flexibility: The main goal of yoga poses is to increase the range of motion and flexibility in the joints while lowering muscle tension and stiffness. Seniors with sciatica may move more easily and effectively with greater flexibility, which lowers the chance of exacerbating their symptoms.

3. Stress Reduction and Relaxation: Adding mindful breathing exercises and meditation to yoga poses helps practitioners feel less stressed, anxious, and tense while also encouraging relaxation and overall well-being. Lower levels of stress can release tense muscles and ease sciatic discomfort.

4. Enhanced Body Awareness: Seniors who practice yoga are better able to tune into their bodies and identify pain or discomfort because it fosters a greater sense of mindfulness and body awareness. People can adjust their practice to prevent worsening their sciatica and move more comfortably and easily by becoming more aware of their bodies.

Tai Chi for Sciatica Relief

Tai Chi is a mild form of martial arts that emphasizes breathing deliberately and moving slowly to improve balance, coordination, and relaxation. Tai Chi, also called "moving meditation," is useful for people of all ages and fitness levels, but it's especially helpful for elderly people who are coping with sciatica.

Tai Chi's advantages for seniors with sciatica

1. Enhanced Balance and Stability: Tai Chi exercises that focus on balancing, controlling movement, and shifting weight can benefit seniors with their balance and stability. Better balance lowers the chance of falls and injuries, which is crucial for people with sciatica because they may feel weakness or numbness in their legs.

2. Stress Reduction and Mental Well-Being: Tai chi combines mindfulness and meditation techniques that encourage calmness, lower stress levels, and improve concentration and mental clarity. Tai Chi has relaxing benefits that can help seniors with sciatica feel more emotionally and mentally at ease.

3. Low-Impact Exercise: Seniors with sciatica or other musculoskeletal disorders can benefit from Tai Chi because it is a low-impact exercise that is easy on the joints and muscles. Tai Chi's deliberate, slow motions increase muscle strength, range of motion, and flexibility without putting undue strain on the body.

4. Pain management: Research has indicated that Tai Chi is beneficial in lowering persistent pain, especially pain brought on by ailments like sciatica. Tai Chi's slow, repetitive motions encourage blood flow and relaxation, which helps people with sciatica feel less tense and uncomfortable in their muscles.

For seniors with sciatica, adding Tai Chi and mild yoga to a regular fitness regimen might be quite beneficial. These mindful movement exercises provide mild strengthening, stretching, and relaxing methods that increase flexibility, reduce discomfort, and improve general well-being. Seniors who regularly practice gentle yoga and Tai Chi can experience relief from sciatic pain as well as increased comfort and mobility in their daily lives.

Tai chi and yoga exercise for seniors with sciatica:

➢ *Five minutes of warm-up*
   1. Neck rolls: Turn your head gently five times in a clockwise and five counterclockwise direction.
   2. Arm circles: Five times in each direction, make little circles with your arms moving forward and backward.
   3. Ankle circles: Make ten rotations of your ankles in each direction, clockwise and counterclockwise.

Yoga for fifteen minutes

1. Cat-cow:

➜ Place your hands shoulder-width apart and your knees hip-width apart as you begin on all fours.

➜ Take a deep breath, arch your back, and lower your belly to the floor, assuming the cow stance.

➜ Exhale, turn your back and adopt the cat stance by tucking your chin into your chest.

➜ Five to ten times over.

2. Seated spinal twist:

➜ Place your hands on your thighs and your feet flat on the floor while you sit in a chair.

➜ Breathe in and glance over your right shoulder as you slowly rotate your upper body to the right.

➜ For a deeper stretch, exhale and lightly place your left hand (palm) against your right leg.

➜ Take a breath and come back to the center position. Continue on the opposite side.

Perform five to ten reps on each side.

3. Modified downward-facing dog position:

➜ Place your hands shoulder-width apart and your feet hip-width apart.

➜ As you walk your hands forward to form an inverted V with your body, hinge at your hips and stretch your spine.

➜ Maintain a slight bend in your knees and press your heels into the ground.

➜ For five to ten breaths, hold.

4. Child Pose

➜ In the child's position, place your toes together on the floor and sit back on your heels.

➜ Put your arms out in front of you and place your forehead down on the ground.

➜ Hold for a duration of 30 to 60 seconds.

Tai Chi for fifteen minutes

1. Cloud hands: Place your knees slightly bent and your feet shoulder-width apart. Let your arms and shoulders drop, and visualize using your hands to gently push clouds away from you. Make wide, fluid movements with your hands.

2. Single whip: Place your knees slightly bent and your feet shoulder-width apart. With your palm facing down, extend your right arm shoulder height in front of you. With a flick of the wrist, imagine that you are holding a whip and cracking it. Continue on the opposite side.

3. Spreading its wings, the wild goose stands with its arms by its sides and feet shoulder-width apart. To mimic a bird spreading its wings, extend your arms out to the sides. After that, reassemble your arms in front of you. Five to ten times over.

5-minute cool-down

To practice deep breathing, find a comfortable posture to sit or lie down, then close your eyes. Breathe in through your nose and out through your mouth slowly and deeply. Breathe deeply and let your body unwind.

---

1. Pay attention to your body's signals and cease any workout that hurts.
2. Adjust the workouts to suit your talents and degree of fitness as necessary.
3. Breathe softly and deeply while performing the exercises.
4. Pay attention to moving mindfully and with a goal.

CHAPTER SIX

EXERCISES FOR BALANCE AND STABILITY

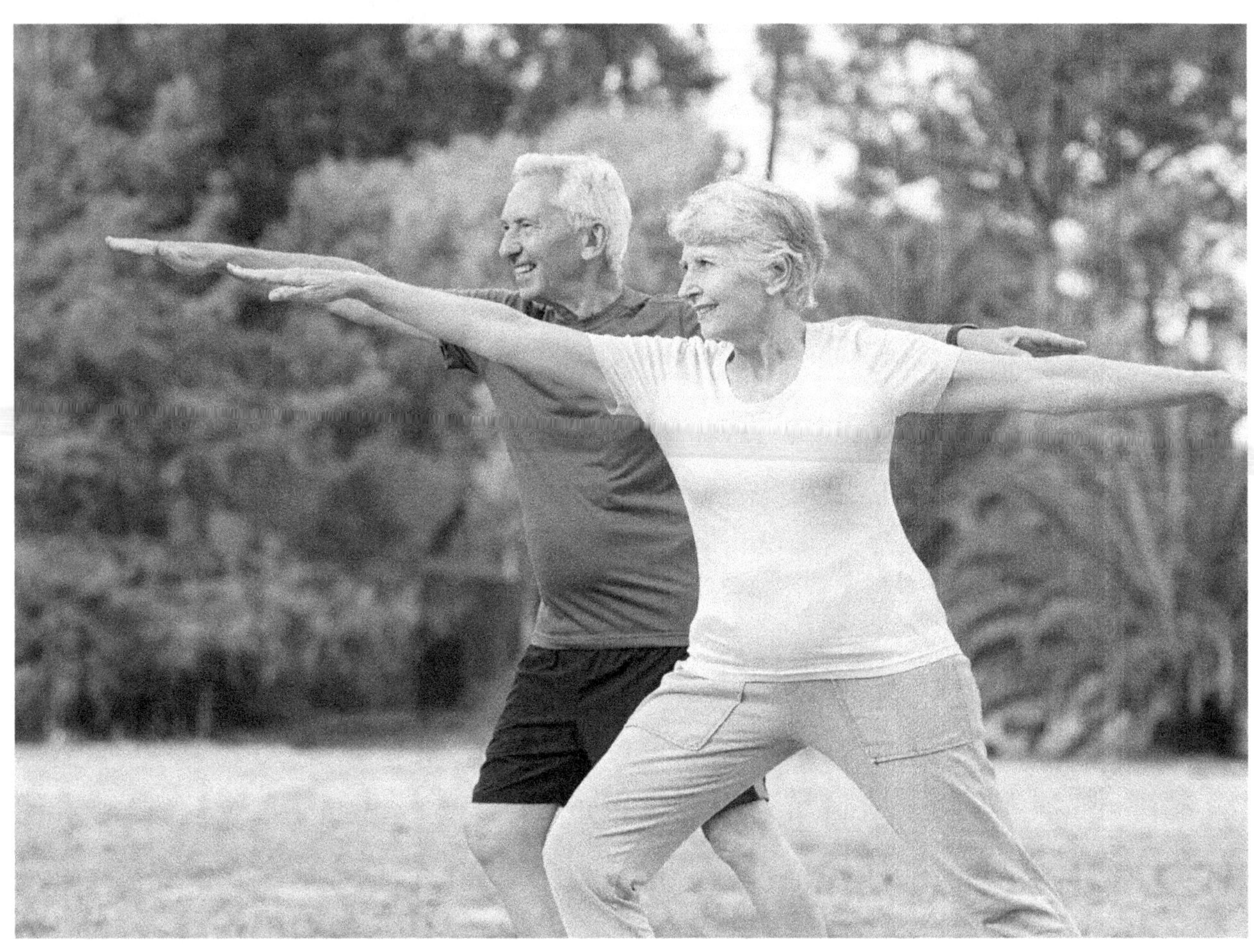

The Importance of Stability and Balance for Seniors

Seniors who manage sciatica, in particular, need to maintain balance and stability. Age-related changes in sensory perception, muscle strength, and flexibility can raise the risk of falls and accidents. Exercises for balance and stability are crucial for people with sciatica since they lower their chance of falling and enhance their quality of life in general.

1. Fall Prevention: By increasing proprioception, or the awareness of one's body position, and coordination, balance, and stability exercises help lower the risk of falls and the injuries they cause. Seniors who suffer from sciatica are more likely to fall because of leg discomfort, numbness, or weakening of their muscles. Seniors can carry out daily tasks more securely and confidently by increasing their balance and stability.

2. Enhanced Mobility: Walking, climbing stairs, and getting in and out of chairs are just a few of the everyday actions that require maintaining balance and stability. Seniors with sciatica benefit from balance exercises because they increase proprioception, joint flexibility, and muscle strength.

3. Lower Risk of Injury: Proper body mechanics and alignment are supported by strong balance and stability, which lowers the risk of musculoskeletal problems. Muscle imbalances or compensatory movements in seniors with sciatica may raise their risk of strain or overuse injuries. Exercises for balance aid in addressing these imbalances and encourage safe movement habits.

4. Better Posture and Alignment: By promoting improved posture and spinal alignment, balance and stability exercises lessen the load on the spine and its supporting tissues. Because of their bad posture or misaligned spines, seniors who suffer from sciatica frequently endure pain or discomfort. Sciatic nerve pressure can be relieved and discomfort can be decreased by strengthening core muscles and enhancing balance.

5. Increased Self-Esteem and General Well-Being: Positivity and general well-being can be enhanced when one feels secure in their capacity to uphold equilibrium and stability. Sciatica sufferers in their senior years may feel scared or anxious about falling or having limited mobility. Regular balancing exercises can foster a sense of mastery

over one's physical talents and help one

gain confidence.

Seniors with sciatica must make balance and stability exercises a daily part of their routine. These activities increase mobility and independence, lower the chance of falling, and improve quality of life in general. Age-related health, safety, and well-being can be preserved by seniors with sciatica by emphasizing balance and stability exercises.

Balance Exercises to Reduce Fall Risk

Exercise 1. Walk on your tiptoes

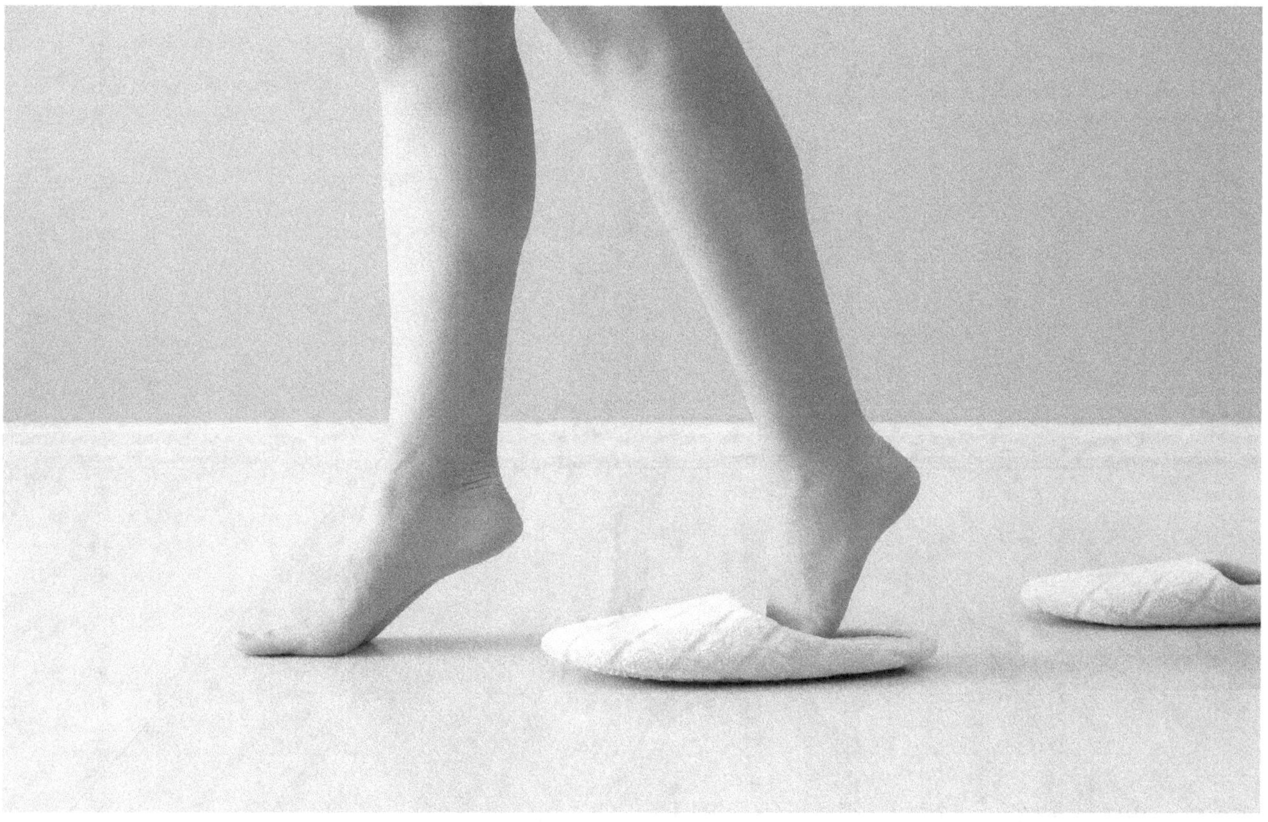

1. With your feet shoulder-width apart and your arms by your sides, start tall.
2. Step forward slowly, keeping the toes of the foot on the inside of the heel of the other foot.
3. Pay close attention to your posture, keep your core strong, and face forward.
4. Ten steps forward should be repeated, followed by a turn and ten steps backward.

Modification

If necessary, use a chair or wall as support.

Without taking your feet off the ground at first, indicate the heel-toe steps.

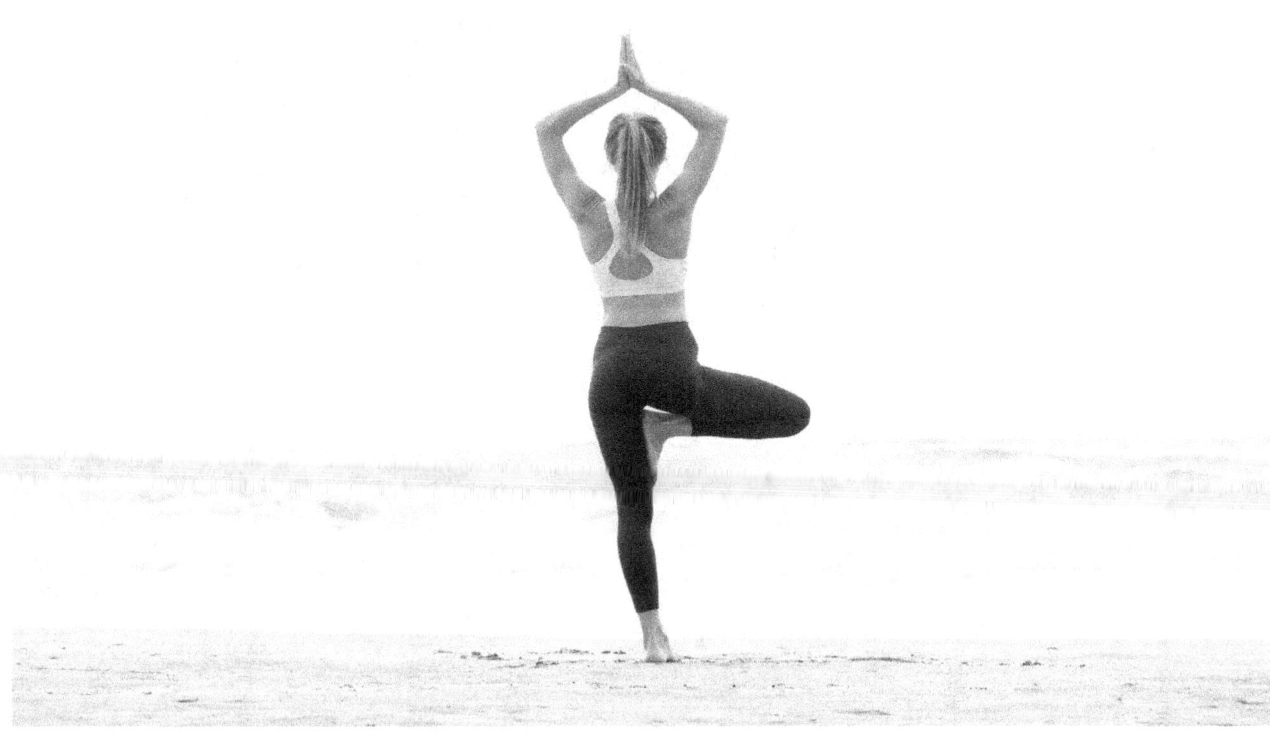

1. Place your feet hip-width apart and stand tall.
2. Lift one leg slowly off the ground and hold it there for five to ten seconds while maintaining an upright posture and your gaze forward.
3. Put your foot down again and switch to the other side.
4. Work each leg for three sets of five repetitions.

Modification

If necessary, use a chair or wall as support.

If you have trouble balancing on one leg, try tapping your toes off the ground rather than lifting your leg.

Exercise 3. Moving aside:

1. With your arms by your sides and your feet shoulder-width apart, take a proud stance.

2. Small, deliberate steps to the side should be taken slowly while maintaining your balance over your feet and gazing in the direction you're going.

3. Ten steps to the right are repeated, then you turn and take ten steps to the left.

Modification

Mark the side-stepping motions first, without first taking your feet off the ground.

For extra balance, make hand gestures such as waving your arms in the opposite direction of the leg you're walking on.

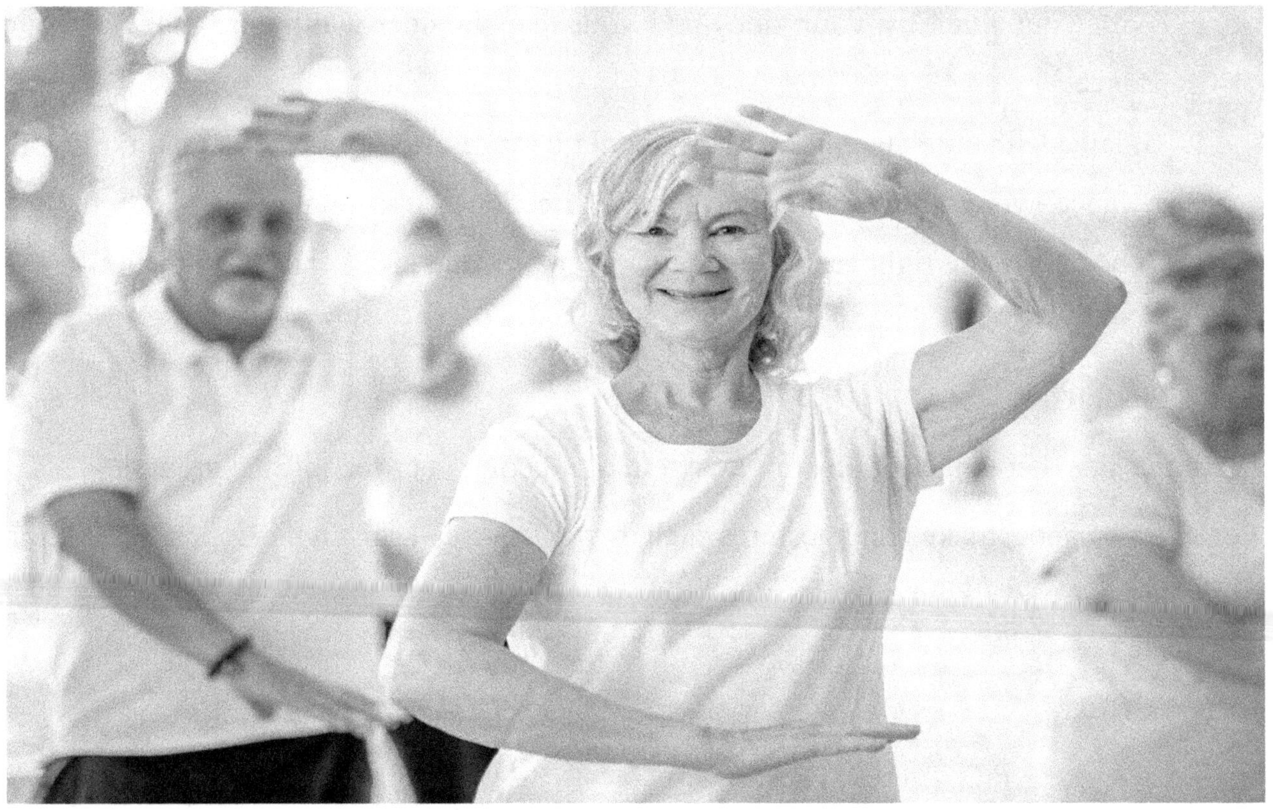

1. With your feet shoulder-width apart and your arms out to the sides, palms down, take a tall stance.
2. While keeping your posture straight and your core active, slowly swing your arms back and forth in a wide arc.
3. Pay attention to how your breath goes with your motions. Take a breath as you swing back and release it as you swing forward.
4. Ten swings in either direction should be repeated.

Modification

If achieving a full range of motion is challenging, use smaller arm swings.

For extra support, grasp onto a chair while you perform the arm swings.

Exercise 5. Reach-based single-leg balance:

1. Place your feet hip-width apart and stand tall.

2. Lift one leg slowly off the ground, and if necessary, grab onto a chair or wall for support.

3. Reach out and touch anything with your free hand, then slowly retract it to your side.

4. On each side, repeat five times.

Modification

If you have trouble balancing on one leg, try tapping your toes off the ground rather than lifting your leg.

If reaching farther is difficult for you, try reaching for your knee or thigh instead of the item in front.

As you gain strength, progressively up the difficulty of the workouts from the beginning.

Pay attention to your body's signals and cease any workout that hurts.

Adjust the workouts to suit your talents and degree of fitness as necessary.

Exercises for Stability to Support the Lower Back

With adjustments for varying ability levels, here are some stability exercises designed to strengthen the lower back and lessen sciatic pain:

Five minutes for warm-up:

1. Neck Rolls: Turn your head gently five times in a clockwise and five counterclockwise direction.
2. Arm Circles: Five times in each direction, make little circles with your arms moving forward and backward.
3. Ankle Circles: Make ten rotations of your ankles in each direction, clockwise and counterclockwise.

Exercises

Exercise 1. Plank:

Begin by placing your forearms parallel to your body and your elbows shoulder-width apart. Form a straight line from your head to your heels by pushing your body up onto your toes. Maintain a flat back and contract your core. Hold for a duration of 15-30 seconds.

Change: For a lower intensity, perform on your knees rather than your toes.

Exercise 2. Dog-bird:

Beginning on all fours, place your hands shoulder-width apart and your knees hip-width apart. Maintaining a flat back and an engaged core, simultaneously extend one arm forward and the opposing leg back. After five seconds of holding, swap sides. Ten repetitions on each side.

Change: Instead of fully extending your knee, perform with it bent and resting on the ground.

Exercise 3. Bridge:

Directions: Place your feet flat on the floor and bend your knees while lying on your back. Squeeze your glutes as you raise your hips off the ground. Hold for five to ten seconds, then gently descend. Ten to fifteen times, repeat.

Modification: If more stability is required, keep one foot flat on the ground.

Exercise 4. Side Board:

Directions: Lie on your side with your forearm flat on the ground and your elbow directly beneath your shoulder. Raise your hips off the floor so that your head and heels are in a straight line. After holding for 15 to 30 seconds, swap sides. For each side, repeat three sets.

Adjustment: To ease the strain, drop your knees to the floor.

For Levels Intermediate/Advanced:

Exercise 5. One-leg deadlift:

Directions: Bend your other leg slightly behind you while standing on one leg. With a flat back and an active core, hinge at the hips and extend your hands downward toward the earth. Resuming your upright position, repeat each side ten times.

Modification: If necessary, use a chair or wall as support.

Exercise 6. bridge of the glutes with a single leg extended:

Steps to follow: 1) Complete the bridge as described above; 2) At the top, raise one leg straight up toward the ceiling. Lower and repeat ten times on each side after holding for three seconds.

Modification:

 If necessary, maintain the extended leg bent at the knee.

Recover (5 minutes):

Main muscle groups should be gently stretched, with each stretch held for 15–30 seconds.

Practice deep breathing.

Increase the number of repetitions and sets gradually at first.

Pay attention to your body's signals and cease any workout that hurts.

CHAPTER SEVEN

CHANGING YOUR LIFESTYLE TO REDUCE SCIATICA

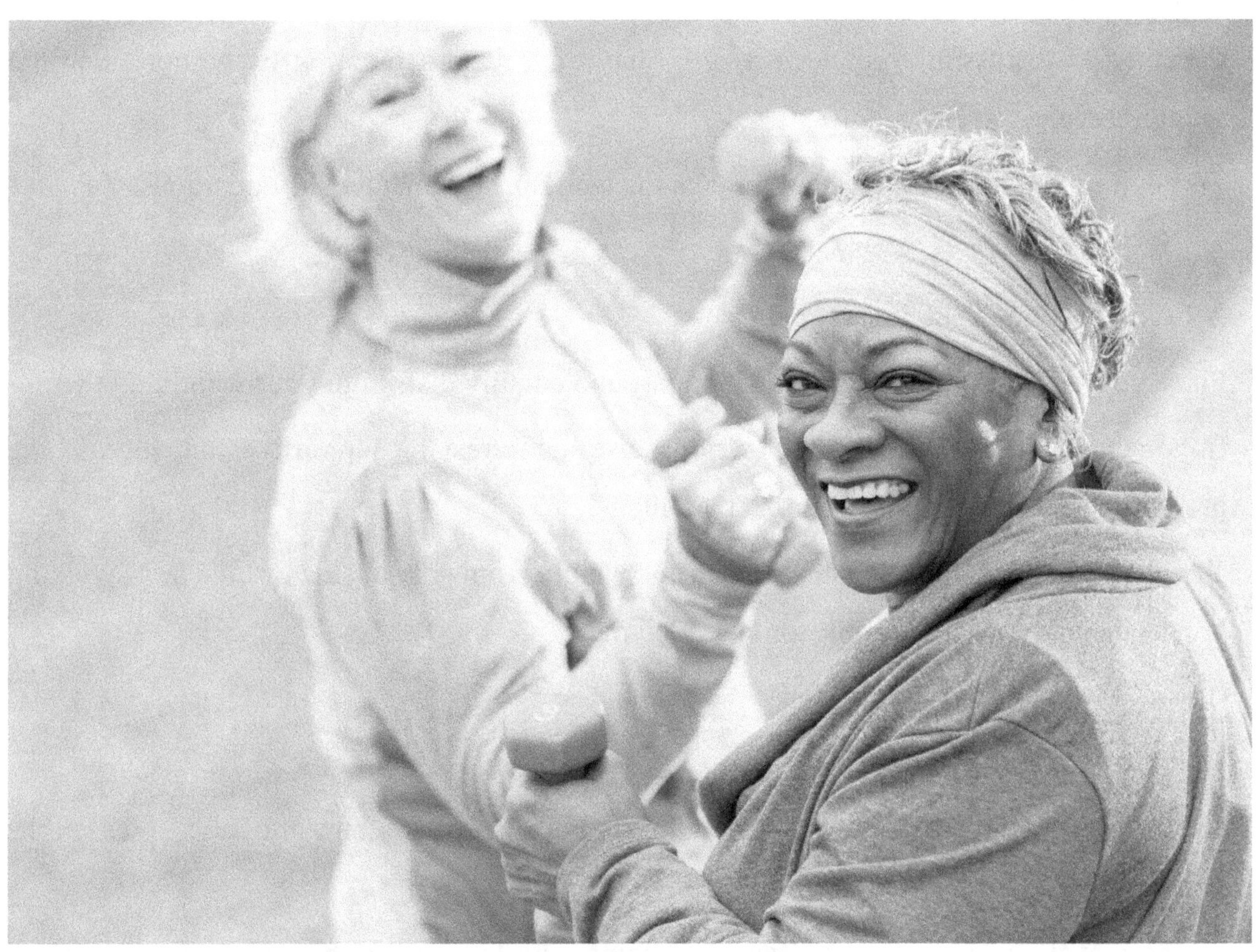

Ergonomic Advice for Typical Tasks

Simple changes to your everyday routine and surroundings can greatly lessen the strain on your spine and ease the symptoms of sciatica. The goal of ergonomic principles is to decrease discomfort and enhance spinal health by maximizing your interaction with your surroundings. The following are some ergonomic pointers for a range of daily tasks:

1. The ergonomics of sitting

Make use of a chair with adequate lumbar support to preserve your lower back's natural curve.

To maintain your knees level with your hips, sit with your feet flat on the ground or supported by a footrest.

Refrain from crossing your legs as this may aggravate symptoms by compressing the sciatic nerve.

Throughout the day, take frequent breaks to stand up, stretch, and shift positions.

2. Ergonomics of Standing:

Place both of your feet shoulder-width apart and equally distribute your weight on them.

If you must stand for extended periods, use a footrest or supportive mat to ease the pressure and exhaustion on your back and legs.

To relieve strain on your spine, move your weight from side to side or take brief walking breaks instead of standing still for extended periods.

3. Taking Up and Transporting:

When carrying large goods, bend your knees and maintain a straight back to lessen the strain on your spine.

Bending at the waist is not as efficient as using your legs to lift objects that are held close to your body.

When lifting or moving large objects, pivot your complete body to change direction rather than twisting your spine.

4. Position of Sleep:

Make sure the mattress you sleep on supports your spine properly; it shouldn't be overly soft or too firm.

Select a pillow that accommodates your neck's natural curve to preserve healthy spinal alignment.

To maintain the alignment of your hips and spine when sleeping on your side, sandwich a cushion between your knees.

To relieve strain on your lower back when sleeping on your back, tuck a small pillow beneath your knees.

5. Motivating Ergonomics:

Position your knees slightly higher than your hips and support your back with the seat of your car to maintain good posture.

If the lower back support offered by your car seat is insufficient, use a lumbar support cushion.

Stretch and relax your muscles frequently throughout lengthy trips, especially if you are in pain or discomfort.

6. Workstation Configuration:

To avoid putting too much strain on your neck and shoulders, position your computer monitor at eye level.

To support your arms and ease the strain on your shoulders and upper back, use a chair with adjustable armrests.

To reduce bending and reaching, keep commonly used things close at hand.

Take quick breaks to stretch and switch positions frequently, particularly if you spend a lot of time at a desk.

These ergonomic recommendations can help you relieve sciatica symptoms, lessen the strain on your spine, and enhance your general comfort and well-being. Always pay attention to what your body tells you, and adjust as necessary to find what suits you best.

Techniques for Correcting Posture

The way one stands has a big impact on the health of the spine and sciatica symptoms. In addition to aggravating sciatic nerve compression, poor posture can also cause pain and discomfort. We will look at practical methods for adjusting posture in this chapter to reduce sciatica symptoms and support spinal health.

Recognizing Appropriate Posture

Maintaining the spine's natural curvature while standing, sitting, and moving is considered proper posture. An essential component of proper posture is:

1. Alignment: When viewed from the side, the head, shoulders, hips, and feet should all be in a straight line.

2. Neutral spine: Preserve the spine's natural curves, with lumbar lordosis (a small inward curve in the lower back), thoracic kyphosis (an outward curve in the upper back), and cervical lordosis (a slight inward curve in the neck).

3. Balance: To prevent putting too much strain on one side of the body when standing or sitting, distribute your body weight equally between both feet.

Techniques for Correcting Posture

1. Mindfulness: Use mindfulness exercises to become more conscious of your posture all day long. Take regular breaks to assess your posture and correct it if necessary.

2. Core Strengthening: Maintaining good posture and spinal alignment can be aided by strengthening the muscles of the abdomen, obliques, and back.

3. Ergonomic Adjustments: To encourage better posture when seated, make ergonomic changes to your workstation, chair, and computer configuration.

4. Stretching and Mobility Exercises: You may support better posture by reducing muscular tension and increasing flexibility by including stretching and mobility exercises in your routine.

5. Posture Braces or Supports: To offer mild reminders to keep correct posture throughout the day, think about utilizing posture braces or supports.

You may progressively correct your posture, lessen the tension on your spine, and get rid of the symptoms associated with sciatica by incorporating these posture correction techniques into your everyday routine.

Tips for Pain Management and Stress Reduction

Although having sciatica can be difficult, there are techniques you can do to lessen your tension and manage your pain. We'll look at practical pain and stress management strategies in this chapter to help you deal with sciatica and enhance your quality of life.

Advice on Managing Pain

1. Heat and Cold Therapy: To lessen pain and inflammation, apply heat or cold packs to the afflicted area.

2. Over-the-counter Pain Relief: Acetaminophen or ibuprofen, two over-the-counter pain medicines, can help reduce mild to moderate sciatica pain.

3. Topical Analgesics: For regional pain relief, apply topical creams or ointments containing lidocaine, menthol, or capsaicin.

4. Physical Therapy: To reduce sciatica symptoms, create a personalized exercise regimen with a physical therapist that focuses on strengthening, stretching, and increasing mobility.

5. Massage Therapy: Consistent massage therapy helps ease sciatic pain, enhance circulation, and lessen muscle stress.

6. Acupuncture: By stimulating particular acupoints in the body, acupuncture may be used as an alternative therapy to help reduce sciatica pain.

How to Reduce Stress

1. Mindfulness Meditation: To lower stress and encourage relaxation, practice mindfulness meditation. Pay attention to your breathing while objectively observing your thoughts.

2. Deep Breathing Exercises: Engage in deep breathing exercises to lower stress levels and trigger the body's relaxation response.

3. Gentle yoga or tai chi exercises can help you relax, release tension in your muscles, and cope with stress.

4. Nature Walks: To lower stress and improve mental health, spend time in nature by going on leisurely walks or engaging in hobbies like birdwatching or gardening.

5. Journaling: You can process stressors and obtain perspective on your experiences by expressing your thoughts and feelings in a journal.

6. Social Support: To share your experiences and get encouragement and validation, reach out to friends, family, or support groups.

You may manage your sciatica and enhance your general well-being by implementing these pain and stress management strategies into your everyday routine.

4-WEEK EXERCISE PLAN FOR SCIATICA RELIEF + FREE GIFTS

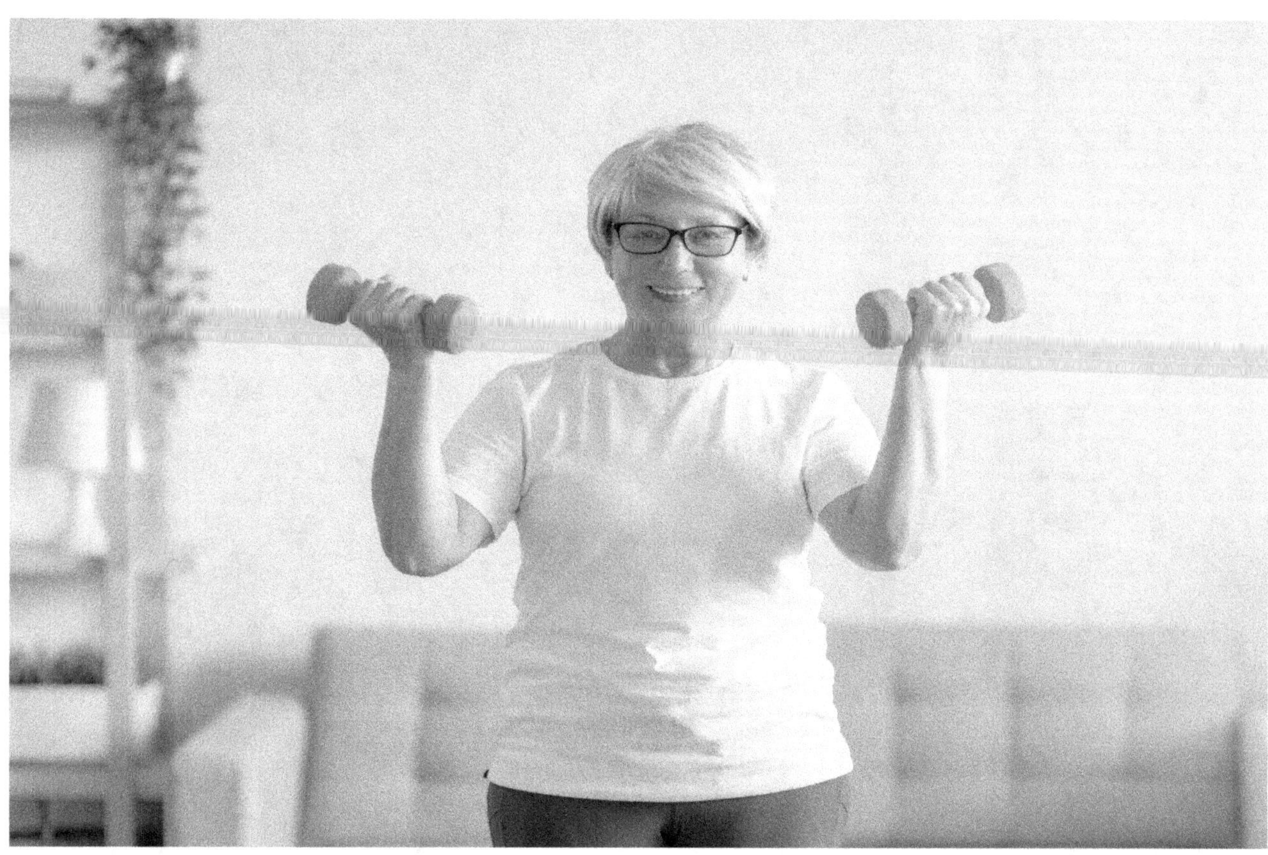

Week 1: Overview of Exercise Program

Day 1–3:

Gentle Cardio: To warm up the muscles and improve blood flow, start with ten to fifteen minutes of low-impact cardio, such as walking or stationary cycling.

Stretching: To increase flexibility and release tension, do a series of mild stretching exercises focusing on the hamstrings, piriformis, and lower back.

Core Activation: To stabilize the spine and promote good posture, activate your core muscles with exercises like pelvic tilts, abdominal bracing, and bird dogs.

Day 4–7:

Rest and Recovery: After introducing exercise to the body for the first time, give it time to recuperate. Make an effort to keep your posture straight and stay active by doing simple things like walking or swimming.

Scan QR Code to Access Video Training

To scan a QR code, take the following general actions:

1. Open the Camera App: The majority of contemporary smartphones come with a built-in QR code scanning feature in their camera apps. Open the camera app on your smartphone.

2. Set the Camera Position: Slightly shake your phone and aim the camera toward the QR code you wish to scan. Verify that the well-lit QR code is inside the frame.

3. Scan the QR Code: The QR code ought to be instantly recognized by your smartphone's camera app. It could provide a link or a notification to access the content linked to the QR code.

4. Follow the Prompt: After the QR code is detected, adhere to any on-screen instructions. This could include clicking on a link to visit a website, downloading an application, or seeing particular content.

5. Access the Content: You ought to be able to view the content linked to the QR code after scanning it and following any instructions. This might be a website, an electronic voucher, contact details, or other kinds of information.

You might need to enable the QR code recognition option in your smartphone's settings or download a QR code scanning app from the app store if the camera app on your phone isn't picking up codes automatically. You should consult your device's user manual for more details since certain devices might have unique motions or instructions for reading QR codes.

Week 2: Increasing Flexibility and Strength

Day 1–3:

Strength Training: To develop strength and stability in the lower body and core, incorporate resistance exercises that target the major muscle groups, such as squats, lunges, bridges, and rows.

Flexibility Training: To preserve flexibility and avoid muscular stiffness, stretch your hamstrings, quadriceps, hip flexors, and glutes after strength training.

Day 4–7:

Cardiovascular Exercise: To enhance cardiovascular health and endurance, extend the time and intensity of cardio workouts to 20–30 minutes. You can use exercises like brisk walking, cycling, or swimming.

Core Strengthening: To challenge core stability and control, add modifications to your core activation activities, like side planks, planks, and stability ball exercises.

Week 3: Increasing Range of Motion and Intensity

Day 1–3:

High-Intensity Interval Training (HIIT): To increase cardiovascular fitness and burn calories, incorporate high-intensity exercise intervals interspersed with active recovery times. Mountain climbers, jumping jacks, and sprint intervals are among the options.

Dynamic Stretching: To enhance the range of motion and prime the body for more strenuous activity, including dynamic stretching movements like arm circles, torso twists, and leg swings.

Day 4–7:

Strength and Balance: To enhance balance, coordination, and proprioception, combine strength training with balancing difficulties like single-leg squats, stability ball exercises, or standing on one leg.

Yoga or Tai Chi: To enhance flexibility, reduce tension, and enhance general well-being, take part in a yoga or Tai Chi practice that emphasizes gentle movements, deep breathing, and relaxation.

Week 4: Maintenance and Consolidation

Day 1–3:

Full-Body Workout: To target numerous muscle groups and maintain overall strength and stability, engage in a full-body strength training program that includes compound movements like deadlifts, push-ups, rows, and overhead presses.

Active recuperation: To encourage recuperation and flexibility without putting undue strain on the joints, partake in low-impact exercises like yoga, cycling, or swimming.

Day 4–7:

Flexibility and Mobility: To preserve flexibility and avoid muscle imbalances, set aside time for stretching and mobility exercises, concentrating on tight or uncomfortable areas.

Mind-Body Connection: To support general well-being and pain management, engage in mindfulness meditation or deep breathing techniques to lower tension, sharpen attention, and increase relaxation.

You can enhance general health and well-being, relieve sciatica symptoms, and progressively increase strength and flexibility by adhering to this 4-week training schedule. Always pay attention to your body, adjust activities as necessary, and see a doctor before beginning a new fitness regimen.

Exercise Planner

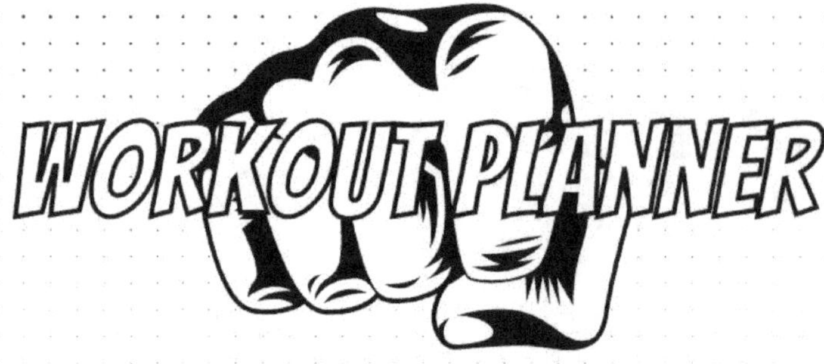

	EXERCISE	GOAL
MON DAY		
TUES DAY		
WEDNES DAY		
THURS DAY		
FRI DAY		

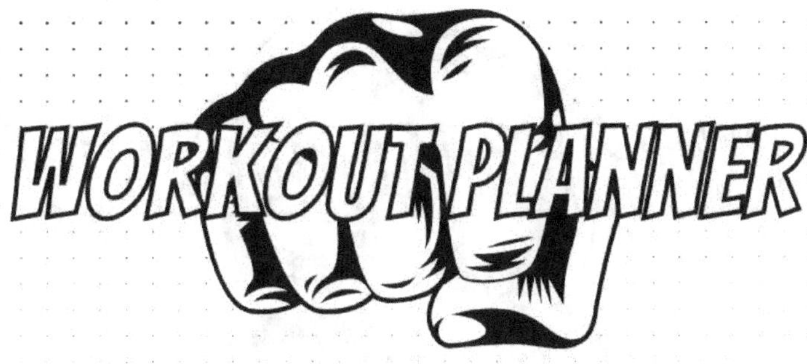

	EXERCISE	GOAL
MON DAY		
TUES DAY		
WEDNES DAY		
THURS DAY		
FRI DAY		

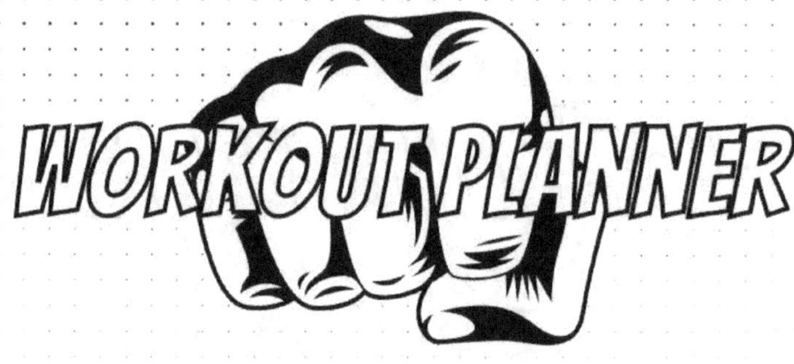

	EXERCISE	GOAL
MON DAY		
TUES DAY		
WEDNES DAY		
THURS DAY		
FRI DAY		

SOPHISTICATED METHODS AND ADVANCEMENTS

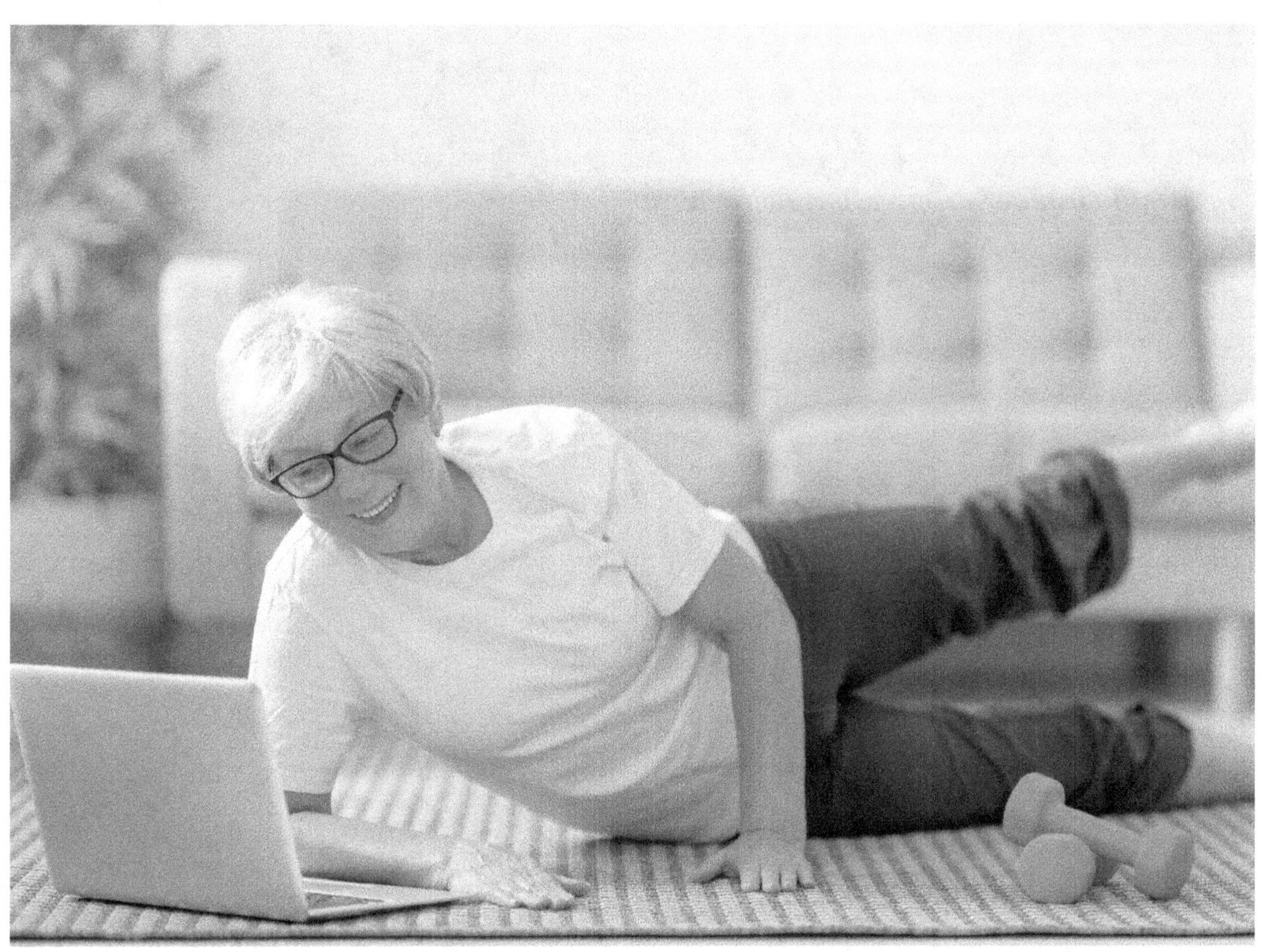

Gradual Increase in Workout Intensity

It's crucial to gradually increase the intensity of your workouts as you go toward better physical health and sciatica treatment. Gradual progression minimizes the chance of damage and maximizes long-term results by enabling your body to adjust to increased demands. To further reduce sciatica symptoms and improve general fitness, we will examine advanced approaches and progressions for progressively increasing exercise intensity in this chapter.

Gradual progression is building up your workouts gradually in terms of frequency, duration, or intensity. You may maintain your gains in strength, flexibility, and endurance while lowering your chance of overuse injuries or setbacks by progressively pushing your muscles, cardiovascular system, and nervous system.

Important Gradual Progression Principles:

1. Start Gradually: Set off at a pace that is comfortable and achievable for your current level of fitness. Before stepping up the intensity, concentrate on perfecting form and technique.

2. Increases Should Be Made Gradually: Raise your workouts' frequency, duration, or intensity by modest percentages every one to two weeks. These increases should usually be between five and ten percent. This keeps your body from overtaxing itself and enables a gradual adaptation.

3. Listen to Your Body: Be aware of how your body reacts to exercise and modify the volume or intensity as necessary. Reduce the intensity or take extra rest days if necessary if you feel pain or discomfort.

4. Periodization: Put periodization strategies into practice by breaking up your training into several periods, like recuperation, strength, and endurance. In addition to optimizing performance and lowering the possibility of overtraining, this enables systematic variation in the training stimuli.

5. Rest and Recovery: Give rest and recovery days top priority so that your body has time to heal and adjust to the strain of exercise. Include active recovery exercises to increase

circulation and lessen discomfort in your muscles, such as yoga, walking, or mild stretching.

More Complex Methods of Gradual Progression:

1. Progressive Overload: To keep your muscles challenged and encourage growth, progressively increase the resistance, repetitions, or sets of strength training exercises.

2. Interval Training: To increase cardiovascular fitness and endurance while optimizing calorie burn, incorporate shorter bursts of higher-intensity activity interspersed with recuperation periods.

3. Complex Training: To increase explosiveness, speed, and agility while enhancing neuromuscular coordination, combine strength and power exercises with plyometric movements.

4. Training volume can be manipulated by changing the quantity of sets, repetitions, or exercises done during a session to gradually increase workload and promote muscle adaptation.

5. Periodization Models: To systematically change training variables and improve performance over time, use periodization models like linear, undulating, or block periodization.

You can effectively manage your sciatica symptoms while making steady progress in strength, flexibility, and endurance by introducing advanced techniques into your training regimen and gradually increasing the intensity of your exercises. When it comes to your fitness regimen, don't forget to prioritize perfect technique, pay attention to your body, and get advice from a qualified trainer or healthcare provider.

Advanced Workouts For Strength and Stability:

1. Single-leg Romanian Deadlift: Hinge at the hips while maintaining a straight back and a tight core. Stand on one leg and grasp dumbbells or weights. When you feel a strain in your hamstrings, lower the weights toward the floor and stand back up. Continue with the opposite leg.

2. Weighted Walking Lunges: Do walking lunges while holding dumbbells or donning weighted ankle cuffs. Leaning forward with one leg, bend both knees to a ninety-degree angle. Repeat with the second leg, pushing yourself back up to the starting position.

3. Press against rotation by lying on your back with your knees bent and your feet flat on the ground. Place a medicine ball or weight against your chest. Lift one leg and your upper body off the ground simultaneously, maintaining a neutral spine and an engaged core. Reverse the process and lower yourself back down.

4. Bosu Ball Plank: With your hands or forearms on the platform side, perform a plank on a Bosu ball. This makes maintaining your core stability much more difficult.

5. Standing on one leg, elevate the other leg slightly behind you to achieve single-leg balance with overhead reach. Take a few seconds to hold one arm raised toward the ceiling. Continue on the opposite side.

6. Star Plank: Form the shape of a star with your arms and legs extended out from the plank posture. As long as you can keep your form correct, hold.

Extra Advice:

If you want an even greater challenge, think about adding resistance bands.

Pay attention to complicated workouts that work for several muscle groups at once.

To keep things fresh and difficult, mix up your regimen.

For a well-rounded workout, combine flexibility exercises with strength training.

Recall that consistency is essential! Frequent exercise enhances strength, stability, and general well-being; however, before beginning any new program, always put safety first and speak with your doctor.

Including Light Weights and Resistance Bands in Your Exercises

Resistance Bands:

1. Boost Intensity: To existing exercises like squats, lunges, rows, and overhead presses, add resistance bands. Depending on the workout, loop the band around your hands, knees, ankles, or legs. When you gain strength, go for a band with more resistance.
2. Target Specific Muscles: For isolation exercises such as lateral raises, tricep extensions, and bicep curls, use loop bands. For stability, fasten the band to a pole or wrap it over a door handle.
3. Incorporate Dynamic Exercises: Employ bands to perform dynamic warm-ups and stretches such as band walks, arm circles, and leg swings. They increase movement and provide controlled resistance.

Try single-leg band exercises, such as standing or single-leg deadlifts, to test your balance. The band adds a challenge to balance while offering support.

Lightweights:

1. Start Gradually: Start with weights that you can lift comfortably ten to fifteen times while maintaining flawless form. Increase weight gradually as your strength increases.
2. Compound workouts: For multi-joint workouts such as squats, lunges, rows, pushes, and deadlifts, use dumbbells or kettlebells. These provide an effective workout by targeting several muscle groups.
3. Exercises for Isolation: For focused exercises like bicep curls, tricep extensions, and shoulder raises, use dumbbells. Several particular muscles to facilitate targeted development.
4. Functional Movements: Make use of weights to perform workouts that replicate commonplace tasks, such as kettlebell swings that simulate picking up objects or overhead lifts that simulate lifting groceries.

Try weighted single-leg exercises like dumbbell lunges or single-arm rows to improve your balance and stability. They strengthen the core muscles and enhance equilibrium.

Blending the Two:

Combination workouts: For workouts like weighted lunges with a band around your knees, overhead presses with resistance bands wrapped around your hands, and light dumbbells in each hand, use both resistance bands and light weights.

Warm-up with Bands, Strengthen with Weights: For dynamic stretches and warm-up, use resistance bands. For strength training, switch to utilizing lighter weights.

Pay Attention to Different Phases: Use weights for low-rep workouts to develop strength and bands for high-rep activities to increase endurance.

Overall Advice:

To prevent injury, concentrate on using weights and resistance bands with good form.

Throughout every exercise, keep your posture straight and use your core.

Breathe regularly and deeply during your exercise.

When your body tells you to take a day off, do so.

Before beginning any new fitness regimen, especially if you have any health issues, speak with a healthcare provider.

Your workout regimen will be more effective if you use resistance bands and modest weights to add variety and push your muscles in new ways. For best results, always start slowly, focus on good form, and pay attention to your body.

CHAPTER NINE

DESIGNING AN INDIVIDUALIZED
WORKOUT ROUTINE

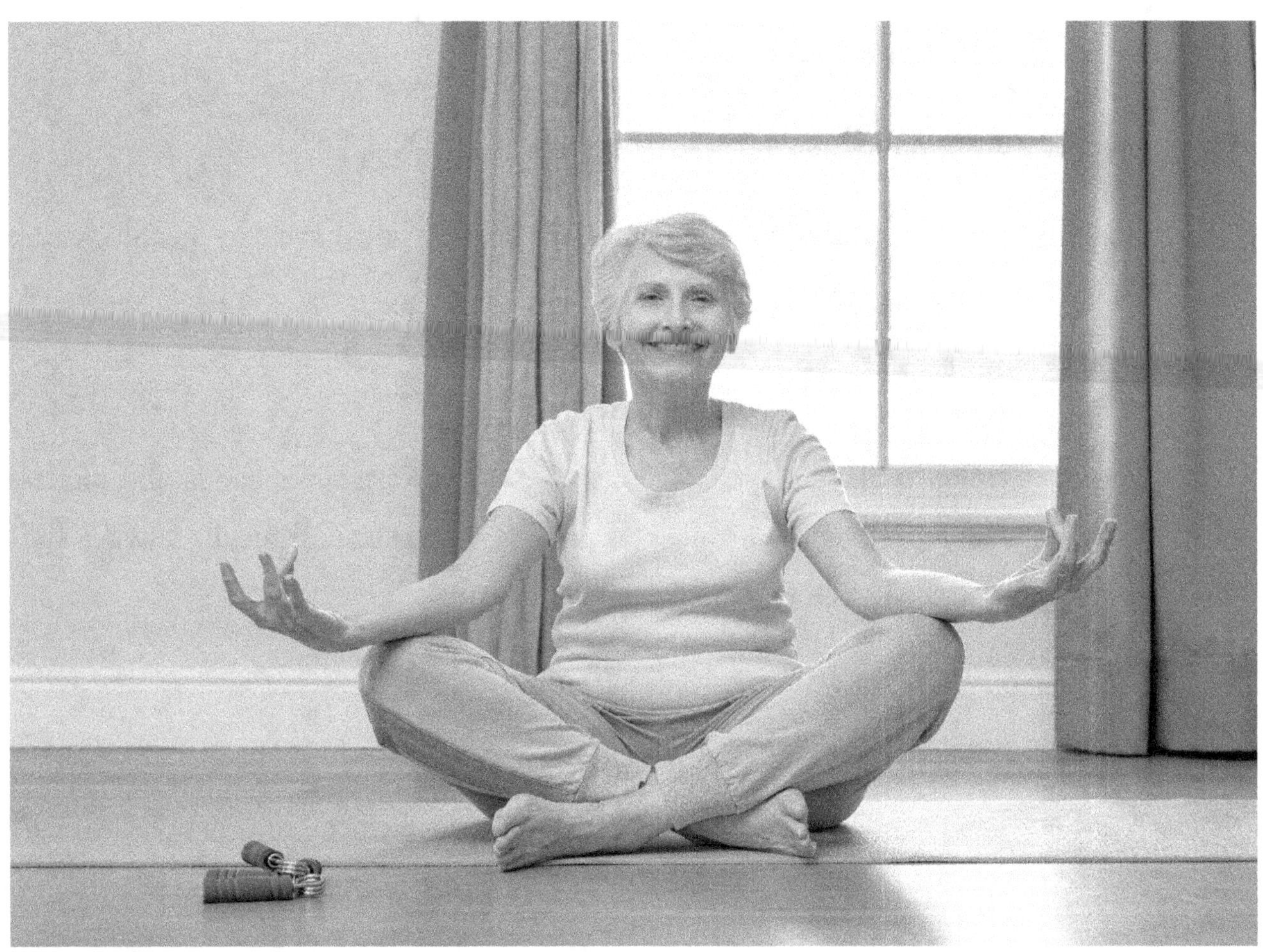

Evaluating Personal Fitness Levels

It's important to determine your exact degree of fitness before starting a customized workout program to relieve sciatica. By evaluating your present level of fitness, you may customize your exercise regimen to meet your unique needs, capabilities, and objectives, enhancing the efficiency of your efforts and lowering your risk of injury. To assist you in creating a personalized exercise regimen for sciatica relief, we will examine a number of techniques for determining an individual's degree of fitness in this chapter.

Recognizing Personal Fitness Elements

Evaluating different physical fitness components, such as the following, is necessary to determine an individual's degree of fitness:

1. Evaluating your respiratory efficiency and cardiovascular endurance, usually through prolonged aerobic activity, is known as cardiorespiratory fitness.

2. Evaluation of your major muscle groups' strength and endurance: This is commonly done by performing activities like push-ups, squats, or weightlifting.

3. Flexibility: The ability to move freely in your joints and muscles; measured using a variety of flexibility tests or exercises that concentrate on specific muscle groups.

4. Assessing the ratio of lean body mass to body fat, or body composition, is done by using measurements such as the body mass index (BMI), body fat percentage, or waist-to-hip ratio.

Techniques for Determining Personal Fitness Levels:

1. Functional Movement Screening (FMS): FMS is a thorough evaluation of basic movement patterns and asymmetries that provide information on areas of imbalance or weakness that may raise the risk of injury.

2. Cardiovascular Fitness Tests: The 1-mile walk test, the 6-minute walk test, and the Rockport Fitness Walking Test are popular tests that evaluate aerobic capacity and cardiovascular endurance.

3. Tests of Strength and Endurance: To gauge your muscles' strength and endurance across a range of muscle groups, try activities like push-ups, squats, lunges, and planks.

4. Flexibility Assessments: To assess range of motion and pinpoint tight or restricted areas, do flexibility tests such as the sit-and-reach test, shoulder flexibility test, or hip flexor test.

5. Body Composition Analysis: To evaluate body composition and ascertain body fat %, use techniques including dual-energy X-ray absorptiometry (DEXA) scans, skinfold caliper measures, and bioelectrical impedance analysis (BIA).

Creating a Customized Workout Program

After determining your level of fitness, you can create an exercise program that is unique to your requirements, tastes, and objectives. Cardiovascular, strength, flexibility, and mobility exercises should all be included in your workout regimen, with the complexity and intensity of the exercises increasing with time. To help you create a safe and efficient exercise regimen that meets your specific demands and supports your journey towards sciatica relief and enhanced general well-being, speak with a licensed fitness expert or physical therapist.

Developing a customized workout regimen is crucial for controlling sciatica and enhancing general health and well-being. It is possible to address the underlying causes of sciatica, strengthen supporting muscles, increase flexibility, and lessen pain and suffering by customizing your exercise regimen to your unique needs, talents, and goals.

Evaluation of Personal Needs and Capabilities

It's critical to evaluate your unique needs, capabilities, and constraints before creating a personalized fitness program. Take into account the following elements:

1. present Fitness Level: Assess your present level of physical fitness, taking into account your flexibility, balance, muscular strength and endurance, and cardiovascular endurance.

2. Medical History: Consider any past operations, illnesses, or injuries that may affect how safely you can exercise.

3. Sciatica Symptoms: Evaluate your sciatica symptoms, such as pain intensity, range of motion, and functional restrictions, as well as their frequency and severity.

4. Personal Objectives: Determine your unique objectives for sciatica alleviation and general health, such as pain reduction, increased mobility, or improved quality of life.

Elements of a Tailored Workout Plan

The following elements of your personalized fitness program might be included, depending on your assessment:

1. Cardiovascular Exercise: To enhance cardiovascular health and stimulate circulation without aggravating sciatica symptoms, use low-impact aerobic exercises like walking, swimming, cycling, or utilizing an elliptical machine.

2. Strength Training: To increase muscular strength, stability, and support for the spine, use resistance exercises that focus on the major muscle groups, especially the lower body, hips, and core.

3. Flexibility and Mobility: To increase flexibility, lessen muscular tension, and relieve pressure on the sciatic nerve, incorporate foam rolling, mobility, and stretching activities.

4. Balance and Stability: To improve proprioception, coordination, and postural control and lower the risk of falls and accidents, including balance and stability exercises.

5. Functional Movement Patterns: To improve movement mechanics and increase functional capacity in daily activities, concentrate on functional movement patterns including squats, lunges, bending, and twisting.

Advancement and Alteration

It's critical to keep an eye on your symptoms as you advance through your personalized workout program and modify your regimen as necessary. Over time, progressively escalate the level of difficulty, duration, and intensity of your workouts to keep your body challenged and encourage adaptation. Furthermore, be ready to adjust your program as necessary if your symptoms, capabilities, or objectives change.

Achieving Practical Objectives for Sciatica Relief

To effectively manage sciatica and maintain motivation during your recuperation process, you must set reasonable goals. You may monitor your development, acknowledge your accomplishments, and keep your attention on your long-term health and well-being by setting specific, attainable goals. We'll talk about practical goal-setting techniques for sciatica alleviation in this chapter.

Setting Particular Objectives

Be clear and quantifiable when establishing goals for sciatica alleviation. Take into account the following elements:

1. Pain Reduction: Establish objectives to lessen the frequency, severity, and length of sciatica symptoms. Some examples of these objectives include a target % reduction in pain or a reduction in the amount of pain medication required.

2. Enhancing Function: Set objectives about enhancing functional capacities and mobility, such as reaching particular movement benchmarks, extending one's range of motion, or reducing discomfort while carrying out daily tasks.

3. Increasing Fitness: To promote general health and well-being, set objectives for increasing physical strength, flexibility, balance, and cardiovascular endurance.

4. Lifestyle Changes: Establish objectives for implementing stress-reduction techniques, proper posture, getting enough sleep, and eating a balanced diet—all of which can help relieve sciatica symptoms.

SMART Objective Establishment

Make sure your objectives are clear, measurable, doable, pertinent, and time-bound by using the SMART criteria:

1. Particular: Clearly state your goals, their significance, and your plan of action.

2. Measurable: Use tools like pain measures, mobility evaluations, or fitness tests to set precise benchmarks for tracking development and achievement.

3. Achievable: Determine tough but doable objectives based on your present skills, available resources, and available time.

4. Relevant: Make sure your aims for sciatica treatment and general well-being are in line with your values, priorities, and long-term ambitions.

5. Time-bound: Establish a deadline for accomplishing your objectives and divide them into more manageable benchmarks or goals to monitor your progress.

Tracking and Modifying Objectives

Track your progress toward your objectives regularly, noting your accomplishments and pinpointing areas that need work. Be adaptable and ready to modify your objectives if your circumstances, abilities, or symptoms change. Recall that obstacles are an inherent aspect of the process, and seize the chance to gain knowledge, adjust, and realign your endeavors.

You can effectively manage symptoms, increase function, and improve overall well-being by designing an exercise program that is specific to your requirements and skills and setting realistic goals for sciatica relief.

CONCLUSION

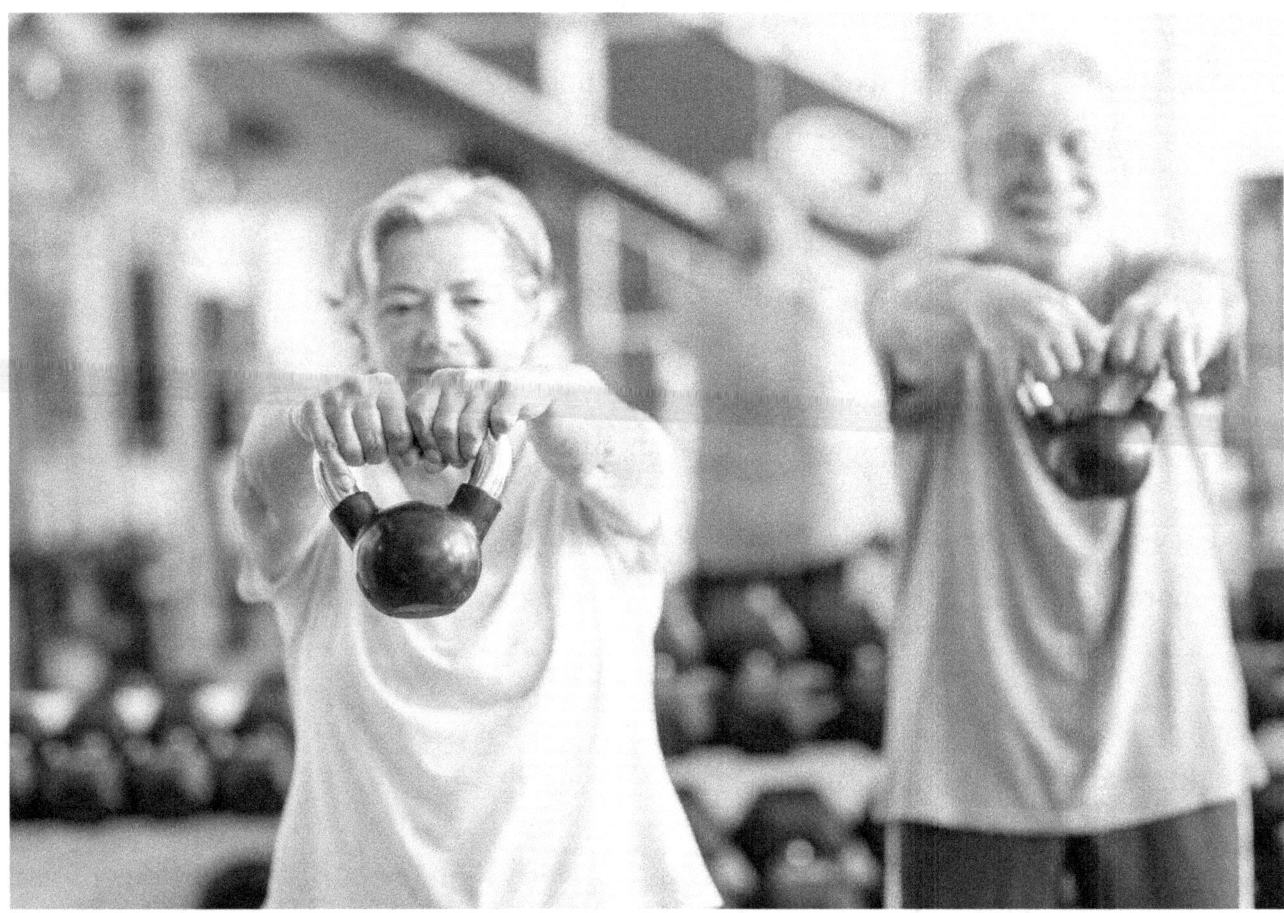

In summary, treating sciatica with a focused exercise regimen provides a way to alleviate symptoms and enhance the quality of life for those dealing with this difficult illness. We've covered a lot of ground in this article on sciatica relief, from diagnosing the illness to creating individualized workout regimens and establishing reasonable objectives. Let's review the main ideas we covered and extend our encouragement for ongoing fitness and wellness as we come to a close.

Recap of Key Points

1. Knowing Sciatica: Sciatica is a disorder that usually results from irritation or compression of the sciatic nerve. It is characterized by pain, tingling, or numbness radiating along the nerve.
2. Importance of Exercise: By enhancing flexibility, lowering pain and suffering, and strengthening supporting muscles, exercise is essential for controlling sciatica.
3. Elements of a complete activity Program: Cardiovascular activity, strength training, work on flexibility and mobility, balance and stability exercises, and functional movement patterns are all part of a complete exercise program for sciatica relief.
4. Setting Realistic Goals: To stay motivated and monitor your progress toward sciatica relief, you must set specified, measurable, attainable, relevant, and time-bound (SMART) goals.
5. Gradual Progression and Modification: The secret to long-term success is to gradually increase the complexity and intensity of your workouts while paying attention to your body and making necessary adjustments to your program.

Encouragement for Continued Exercise and Wellness

Remember that perseverance and consistency are essential when you set out on your path to better health and sciatica treatment. Accept the process of making incremental progress over time, rejoice in your little accomplishments, and don't let failure depress you. Your commitment to self-care and regular exercise will pay off in the shape of improved mobility, less discomfort, and general health.

Remember that your fitness regimen is only one part of your journey toward total well-being. Including healthy lifestyle practices like stress reduction, appropriate sleep, good eating, and frequent activity throughout the day will help you achieve sciatica relief and the best possible health.

Lastly, keep in mind that you are not traveling alone. Consult medical specialists, fitness instructors, or support groups for direction, accountability, and encouragement. Sciatica can be well managed and you can lead an active, fulfilling life if you have endurance, drive, and a commitment to your health.

My best wishes to you as you continue to pursue optimal health and relief from sciatica!

Scan QR Code to Access Video Training

To scan a QR code, take the following general actions:

1. Open the Camera App: The majority of contemporary smartphones come with a built-in QR code scanning feature in their camera apps. Open the camera app on your smartphone.

2. Set the Camera Position: Slightly shake your phone and aim the camera toward the QR code you wish to scan. Verify that the well-lit QR code is inside the frame.

3. Scan the QR Code: The QR code ought to be instantly recognized by your smartphone's camera app. It could provide a link or a notification to access the content linked to the QR code.

4. Follow the Prompt: After the QR code is detected, adhere to any on-screen instructions. This could include clicking on a link to visit a website, downloading an application, or seeing particular content.

5. Access the Content : You ought to be able to view the content linked to the QR code after scanning it and following any instructions. This might be a website, an electronic voucher, contact details, or other kinds of information.

You might need to enable the QR code recognition option in your smartphone's settings or download a QR code scanning app from the app store if the camera app on your phone isn't picking up codes automatically. You should consult your device's user manual for more details since certain devices might have unique motions or instructions for reading QR codes.